Residents

The Perils and Promise of Educating Young Doctors

DAVID EWING DUNCAN

SCRIBNER

SCRIBNER
1230 Avenue of the Americas
New York, NY 10020

SCRIBNER *and design are*
trademarks of Simon & Schuster Inc.

Set in Adobe Trump Medieval
Designed by Jenny Dossin

Manufactured in the United States of America
1 3 5 7 9 10 8 6 4 2

Library of Congress Cataloging-in-Publication Data is available.
ISBN 0-684-19709-X

To LRD,
and to all residents, past, present, and future

There is this system that essentially was started by this visionary, William Osler, just before the turn of the century. And that basic system has not changed in a hundred years despite tremendous changes that have gone on in American medicine. The mandate now is for substantial change, to fundamentally restructure the way we teach physicians.

John Stobo, M.D., Chief of Medicine,
Johns Hopkins Hospital, 1985–1995

AUTHOR'S NOTE

Where subjects have asked me to keep their names anonymous, I have used pseudonyms and made minor changes. None of these alterations have materially affected the essential facts as I observed or heard them. At times dialogue has been edited and condensed and in some cases resequenced to avoid unnecessarily repetitious or irrelevant material.

Like the army, teaching hospitals have developed a system of ranks and titles one needs a guide to follow, starting with the term *resident*. Once, it referred to a trainee physician who literally lived in a hospital. Today, it is the term used for any postgraduate medical student completing his or her clinical requirement to be licensed as a physician, and to be certified to practice a medical specialty. Other ranks, titles and terms:

Intern: a first-year resident. Also called a PGY1 (Post Graduate Year 1); or R1 (Resident [Year] 1).

Junior resident: a second-year in internal medicine, and a second- or third-year in surgery. Also called an R2 or PGY2 in medicine; or an R2 or R3, or a PGY2 or PGY3 in surgery.

Senior resident: a third-year in internal medicine; or a fourth- or fifth-year in surgery. Also called an R3 or PGY3 in medicine; or an R4 or PGY4 in surgery.

Chief resident: In general medicine, the chief resident is a physician who has recently completed a residency, and has been chosen for a year to run the day-to-day operations of the residency program. In surgery, a chief resident is usually a fifth-year resident who serves a similar function, typically overseeing a different group of junior residents each month.

Fellow: A physician who has finished a basic residency and is continuing his or her training to become a specialist.

Residency director: A senior physician permanently assigned to administer the residency program in a given department. He or she organizes the curriculum and handles recruitment.

Chief of service: A senior physician permanently assigned to oversee a department or a section of a department within the hospital, such as the intensive care unit or vascular surgery.

Department chairman: A physician in charge of an entire department, such as surgery, general medicine, pediatrics, or OB–GYN.

Attending: Any licensed physician who has finished his or her residency training, and either admits patients to be cared for by residents, or supervises residents in the hospital.

CONTENTS

A Long, Cold Winter

There is occasions and causes why and wherefore in all things.

William Shakespeare, *King Henry V*

This book originates with a dilemma, and a choice I faced one long, cold winter four years ago. At the time, my wife of six years was fading before my eyes; her skin turning pale, her eyes red-rimmed. Normally cheerful and outgoing, she was losing interest in food, exercise, family, and virtually everything she loved. Six months earlier, she had begun a residency in pediatrics. We knew the training would be tough, with eighty- to one-hundred-hour weeks, overnight shifts up to thirty-six hours every third or fourth night, and an hourly rate paying less than minimum wage. We had friends already undergoing the ordeal, and had watched the circles darken under their eyes. Most were making it, but not all. One friend had seriously contemplated suicide. Two more had had their marriages fail. Yet another, whose career had looked particularly promising, was reprotedly caught stealing a powerful narcotic from his hospital, apparently for his own use.

Our resident friends talked about minor errors and near misses with patients, blamed on fatigue, fear, and inexperience—the surgical intern falling asleep on her feet in the operating room; the junior surgeon left to perform one of his first open heart massages unsupervised; the PGY2 (Post Graduate Year 2) who added an extra zero to a dosage of insulin, caught only at the last minute by the nurse injecting the drug into the patient's intravenous line. Now and then, we would hear about the thrill of puzzling out a diagnosis or saving a life—the deep satisfaction of running a complex regimen of drugs that worked, or mastering the subtle turn of a scalpel during a difficult surgery. More often, we worried about friends alternately exhausted, cynical, and stalwart, who gradually took on the dull, tired-to-the bone, just-barely-getting-by demeanor of survivors.

None of this deterred us from believing we would take our own residency experience in stride, even as my wife suddenly found herself one hot July on an infant's ward working ninety-hour weeks and responsible for up to a dozen tiny charges—newborns with malformed hearts, babies with AIDS, babies abused by their parents, babies slowly dying of bacterial infection. In August, she moved to the emergency room, where she worked a progression of night shifts, afternoon shifts, and morning shifts, all in the same week. On balance, she found her work in the hospital stimulating and occasionally breathtaking. But as the weeks wore on, her enthusiasm dimmed against a relentless onslaught of stress and fatigue. She even began to question why she had become a doctor. Five years earlier, she had entered medical school for all the right reasons—because she wanted to help people, particularly children; and to challenge herself intellectually. Now her idealism was being subsumed by what at times seemed a senseless test of endurance.

Hardly a newcomer to stress, my wife had worked on Wall Street as an investment banker before switching to medicine, and had thrived, easily enduring the hours, deadlines, and cutthroat competition. She also is as dedicated, hardworking, and responsible as anyone I know.

As fall turned to winter, and the air grew cold and flakes of snow began to fall, I became frantic. I loved this woman, and she was hurting. By January, I began asking questions of physician and resident friends, and of medical educators I knew, and anyone else who might offer an explanation, fully expecting a profession steeped in science to have a ready and plausible explanation for something as crucial as how physicians are trained in the United States. Sadly, I was mistaken. Indeed, I was stunned when educators defended the rigor and long hours not with data but with homilies about tradition, and assumptions based on a powerful, almost religious faith in the veracity of their system. "This method has produced the best doctors in the world," said one educator. Claiming a "great sensitivity" to his residents' ordeal, he nonetheless resolved that "it has to be this way." Others talked about the residency as an initiation rite, insisting this was a profession where one has to be as tough and unflinching as a soldier in battle. Countering these comments were residents and physicians critical of the system, who told me, sometimes bitterly, that the residency was unduly harsh and too often left residents damaged for life. Some also claimed the residency placed patients at risk far more often than was necessary.

Both replies fed into my growing fear—that there was *no good reason for this*. Still, I hoped these people were wrong, and that a little digging would turn up a compelling reason to satisfy what seemed a reasonable enough query: "Why does it have to be this way?"

This left me one frigid January evening to consider my options—and to make a choice. Should I simply accept what was happening, gritting my teeth and doing nothing, hoping that everything would be all right when my wife finished? Or should I actively pursue the answer to the question "Why?"

Never one to grit my teeth for long, I launched a personal quest in the only way I knew how—as a journalist taught to investigate. I collected studies. I spoke with dozens of residents, medical educators, patients, nurses, orderlies, medical historians, and other assorted experts. I spent time in hospitals following residents on call.* I kept files on residency fatigue, supervision, curriculum, finances, attitudes, and outcomes.

I quickly ascertained that my wife's ordeal was not only common, but apparently accepted as a necessary evil by a large part of the medical community—including educators I knew and respected, who had reputations as excellent physicians and dedicated teachers. Indeed, I saw no evidence that the vast majority of physician-educators were intentionally cruel, as some critics have insinuated. Quite the opposite, I came to believe that most were caring people who would be horrified if they ever thought their methods were hazardous, either to patients or residents.

This left me facing a paradox. How could medical educators be devoted to patients and to tutelage, yet be so seemingly coldhearted to their trainees? It made no sense until I happened on a letter published in the *Journal of the American Medical Association* in 1989, about burnout among young doctors. In it, the author defended the rigors of the modern residency by concluding with a quote:

* "On call" refers to a period of time, usually a day and an overnight, when a resident is assigned to stay in the hospital to admit new patients, take care of patients already admitted, and supervise more junior residents and medical students. Traditionally, a call "day" lasts thirty-six hours, from seven A.M. the first day to roughly seven P.M. the following evening.

We only go around once, and even to consider burnout, you
must first burn [with passion].

I thumbtacked these words above my desk and pondered them,
finally deciding they were true. Certainly, this is the way I prefer to
live, agreeing with Oliver Wendell Holmes (a famous physician as
well as a literary man) that one ignores passion "at peril of being
judged not to have lived." However, there is a great weight of philosophy, literature, and common sense that warns about taking
passion to excess. To "burn with passion" is—or should be—a matter of degree. This is particularly true when the flames are purpose-
fully blown too high. Nor is burnout among residents and other
physicians necessarily good for the patient, particularly if a single
person is made to suffer or is in any way inconvenienced merely so
that a trainee can "burn with passion."

I contend that it's possible to be impassioned *and* well rested,
resolute *and* compassionate. My wife is passionate about medicine.
But she and other physicians I know are also devoted to living a full
life, to being well rounded, complete people. And they are not only
superior doctors for it but, I suspect, are better healers to their
patients, who presumably trust not only their technical skill but
their ability to empathize, to touch, to talk to them like people
instead of mere receptacles of disease.

Like it or not, medicine today requires physicians to be far more
than monastic technocrats or paternalistic, godlike dispensers of
pills and prognoses. They must have a broad knowledge of finance,
ethics, and law. In an age of consumerism and shared decisions
between doctor and patient, they need to be conversant in the arts of
persuasion and diplomacy. More than ever, they are expected to
take a leading role in solving a host of societal problems, from AIDS
and euthanasia to managed care restrictions and the uninsured. Yet
medical education continues to operate largely in a vacuum, where
humanity is often subsumed by science, and educators consider it far
more important for residents to endure ninety- and hundred-hour
weeks in the cloister of the ward or operating room than to learn
about real life.

Polls tell us that Americans more than ever in recent history are
having trouble trusting physicians, with one recent poll ranking
doctors fifth among the least trusted type of worker—after lawyers,

car salesmen, politicians, and garage mechanics. If true, this should send shivers up and down our collective spines. For if any society wants to be healthy, it must trust its healers, a notion that goes back to shamans and witch doctors, and the belief that charms made of rattlesnake tails and alligator teeth could ward off hurricanes and disease.

The current system produces technically proficient doctors. But does it produce healers? Is it safe for patients? Is it the best we can do?

After four years of observing in over a dozen hospitals, living among residents as they work and eat and (occasionally) sleep, amassing thousands of pages of studies and documents, and conducting some two hundred interviews, there is no question in my mind that medical education in the United States is out of step with patients' and society's needs—and too often dangerous. There have been reforms, though lately the pace has slowed. Most residents no longer work every other night on call. Some programs have limited the number of new patients a single resident can admit while on an overnight call. Others now assign a resident to admit patients late at night—a "night float"—so that the residents on call can catch up with their work, or even sleep. In some hospitals, inexperienced residents are more closely watched by senior physicians than in the recent past. Residents are also getting out of the rarefied world of the hospital ward now and then, working month-long stints in outpatient clinics and doctors' offices. Yet as one educator told me in great frustration, these reforms remain "Band-Aids on a bleeder," the bleeder being a system that still overworks residents, exploits them financially as cheap labor, and frequently plunges them into the thick of sick and dying patients with minimal training and guidance—all because this is the way it's been done for decades, and because many educators continue to insist there is no better way to educate physicians.

The system has checks and balances to protect patients. But I will argue on these pages that while these once may have worked, they are now breaking down in an era of rapid change—in knowledge, in technology, and in the structure of a health care system that today hardly resembles what was considered the norm even a decade or two ago. Patients admitted to hospitals are sicker, they stay for a shorter time, and they have much more done to them in terms of treatment. They also are demanding more participation in decisions. So are insurance plans, as managed care rapidly smashes apart the *ancien régime* of medicine, in which physicians reigned supreme, not insurers. Yet we are still teaching physicians essentially the same way we did a century ago, when the modern residency was invented.

For some reading this book, issues such as resident work hours may seem like yesterday's news. "We all know residents get tired," said an editor-colleague of mine in New York. Yes, I said, but the point is that they are *still* tired—and *still* working under conditions that would seem outrageous in any other industry, particularly those in which lives are riding on a human operator or specialist being alert, well-trained, and optimal. Would we tolerate pilots working twenty-four to thirty-six hour shifts with minimal sleep? Once, pilots flying long hours was allowed, and calls for reductions rebuffed. It took a relentless effort over decades to correct the situation and, tragically, numerous crashes.

Likewise, with the sudden advent of managed care, many of the themes and conundrums contained in this book—work hours, supervision, the rise of technology, the role of philosophy and ethics, how to teach the art of medicine—will seem off the mark for those educators and health care analysts whose attention is (understandably) hyper-focused at the moment on the survival of the academic hospital. With neither government nor the private sector willing to pay what they did for education, indigent care, and research, some teaching hospitals are battling for their financial lives. In this book, I outline some of the dilemmas and possibilities posed by this new world order, though I'm saving the larger story of what will happen to academic medical centers for my next book, which will trace the history of a single academic hospital from its roots in the early nineteenth century to the present. The idea is to explain, using stories and profiles of people, where we are and where I think we should be going in designing a health care system that makes sense.

My aim in *Residents* is not to point fingers. Nor is it an effort to cast about for villains or to create a sensation. I am critical of the system, but I understand that most in it are trying their best within the context of a profession that is notoriously slow to change its basic attitudes. I am also not a physician, which means my criticism will be immediately suspect to many who are. Yet I suggest that nonphysicians, with careful study and immersion into the culture of the teaching hospital, have an important point of view, since nonphysician and physician alike benefit or are harmed by the health care system.

Which brings us back to the question I asked during that long, cold winter nearly four years ago. Does the training have to be this way?

On the following pages, I pose what I hope is a reasoned and, in my own way, passionate argument that it does not—writing not as the frustrated spouse of a resident, but hopefully as an investigator amassing what I consider to be compelling proof that the residency system, and how we train our healers, remains in need of serious overhaul. I have done my best to capture the essence of the American residency and of major trends, though it is far beyond the scope of this book to be all-inclusive for a system that right now is training almost 100,000 residents and specialty fellows in 7,200 residency programs at over 1,200 teaching hospitals.

It has been two years since my wife finished her residency. I am relieved to report that the afflictions of her ordeal were temporary. She is back, as if from an extended journey far from home. Our children once more have a mother who is awake, engaging, beautiful, and able somehow to handle a still demanding fellowship and to be there for friends, family, and patients. Best of all, she endured her training without being fundamentally changed for the worse, or permanently losing her idealism about life and medicine. Regrettably, this is not always the case.

This book is written with the understanding that the residency is, and should be, a challenging and, at times, grueling experience. Because lives are at stake, a physician must be dedicated, responsible, and technically proficient. The question is how can we achieve this without needlessly imperiling residents, patients, and society? I ask this not to provoke or titillate, but to suggest that surely we can devise a better way to train America's healers.

31 Hours

Before you can understand anything about what we do,
you have to stay up with us, eat with us, see our patients.
You have to do the overnight call.

Third-year resident

Jim Stern is furious. A sixty-five-year-old cancer patient, Mary Allen, is dying. Bald and emaciated, her bones wrapped in gray skin as thin as tissue paper, she struggles to draw breath as her lungs rapidly fill with fluid. As she fades in and out of consciousness, her eyes every so often snap open in terror and she moans her own death chant: a feeble "No, no, no."

Heroics, says Jim Stern, a general medicine intern, might save Mary for a few more days or weeks. They could drain her lungs again, he says, but "Her prognosis is essentially zero, so there is no point." He talks while rushing down the hall, headed for a phone to try again to reach the woman's family. "She should be DNR," he mutters, angry because he had been too busy that week to secure a "Do Not Resuscitate" order, a legal permission to let a terminal patient die. Without it, Mary Allen waits in a tormented limbo. Jim isn't going to give her a morphine drip to ease her pain without the family's consent. And he is adamantly against siphoning off the rising tide of fluids, which at best might keep her alive—and in pain— a few more days or weeks.

Stern, twenty-eight, is a PGY1 (post graduate year 1), nine months out of medical school and two-thirds finished with the medical boot camp known as internship. Athletic and handsome with close-cropped hair, he is usually easygoing. Tonight he looks harried, his eyes swollen, his face pale as he swigs Coke after Coke, for the caffeine, he says.

Back in Mary Allen's room, Jim discovers the nurse hasn't administered the sedative he had ordered in lieu of morphine. He flashes a stormy look at the nurse, who lamely tells him the patient was "asleep" earlier. Jim asks her tersely to administer .5 milligrams of Ativan. He walks out. Down the hall, at the resident's station, he dials up phone numbers in Mary's thick chart, desperate to tell her family she is dying and must be designated a DNR. He tries sisters, daughters, friends, finally reaching Mary's grandson. Leaving an urgent message to call back, he slams down the receiver. "Is there anything worse than having to talk to a fourteen-year-old on the telephone? He knows something's amiss, and he's probably scared."

Jim is punching in another number when his beeper squawks. "Stern," he says warily, guessing correctly that the emergency room has another admission for him. He jots down particulars. Eighty-seven years old. White. Male. Renal failure. Diabetes. High blood pressure. Flu. Blind. Disoriented. Possible Alzheimer's. Possible pneumonia. Jim asks the intern covering the E.R. to start the man's orders. "I can't do it now," Jim says. "I'm up to my eyeballs." On his clipboard, he adds the patient to the seven already on his roster, plus eighteen more he will cross-cover tonight for the other two interns on his team, Team Alpha.* The list includes two young AIDS patients, three heart attack victims, a thirty-seven-year-old I.V. drug abuser, a twenty-six-year-old elementary school teacher dying of leukemia, two patients with Alzheimer's, and several frail, demented octogenarians Jim says "are here to crash and die."

Beeeeeep! goes Jim's pager again. He runs his fingers through his hair, which he does whenever he is tense. "I'm getting slaughtered," he says. We both look at a clock on the wall: six-thirty-five P.M. Jim has been in the hospital for 11 1/2 hours, since early morning rounds. But his day has hardly begun. As the intern on call, he will be here until tomorrow afternoon, on a call shift he takes every third night. It lasts a day, a night, and the following day, meaning that he is routinely in the hospital for thirty or more hours, and sometimes as many as thirty-six. (Others in Stern's hospital told me they had stayed forty hours or longer on rare occasions.) Tonight he will be virtually alone on his ward, in charge of twenty-five patients. He has backup: second- and third-year residents in the emergency room, interns on other rotations, and an attending or two working in other parts of the hospital, all of whom are as busy as he is. He can also call

*Interns are required to stay overnight in the hospital only when they are on call.

his own senior resident at home—or, if he is really in trouble, the attending physician in charge of his team, though this is seldom done. The point of the training is for Jim Stern to handle everything by himself, calling in help only if all else fails. If he's lucky, he'll snatch an hour or two of sleep.

■

The day began for Stern at seven o'clock, just after dawn, when he walked from his small apartment a few blocks from the hospital to join Team Alpha for morning rounds. I joined him in the lobby, here on the suggestion of a friend who told me I could never understand the residency without experiencing an on-call shift with an intern—all thirty or more hours of it. On my first of many on-call shifts, I could never have imagined as I waited near the busy information desk, standing off to one side from the mayhem of patients, visitors, physicians in green scrubs and starched white coats, a flower delivery person pushing a cart full of roses, and an old man selling newspapers, that virtually everything fascinating and terrible about the modern residency would play itself out over the next thirty-one hours.

Heading up to a small conference room on the fourth floor of the main hospital tower, Jim introduces me to Dr. Frank Luccia, a second-year resident and the team's leader. He is giving his interns that morning's list of twenty-two patients currently on their service. Using a shorthand mostly incomprehensible to a nonphysician, he has written down vitals, diagnoses, and questions to be answered:

TEAM ALPHA

Wentz, L	96y/o M bilat. cataracts, glaucoma s/p fal
456030	Cataract surg (–/9) ?Nursing Home placement
Phil, G	29y/o M, CAH, Cirrhosis, resolving hep encephalopathy, S. pnem.
320009	bacteremia E. coli SBP (ancef –/4, comp –/10)

Blood Cx.	I/O's	lytes:	Wt:
Bun/Cr k	PT		
Dx/Therapeutic Paracenti (–/10)			

Hermone, S.	78 y/o F met. squamous cell lung ca
567412	with FTT
DNR	?Social Service

Luccia next leads the team—three interns and two medical students—on a lightning-quick tour of their patients, skipping stable ones and pausing briefly to say hello to those who are conscious. A small, intense man with oval, rimless glasses, Frank stops here and there to ask the medical students quick questions. "This patient has a fever, so why don't we give him Tylenol?" "Why are we watching this patient's white count?" "Should we be worried about a bilirubin of 14?"

As the day progresses, I take each member of Team Alpha aside and ask them about their training. Jim Stern, who was chosen for me by his department chief, is the most gung ho about his program. "They hold our hands here," he says, ticking off reforms made in recent years—special nursing teams to handle "scut work,"* the switch to an every third night call schedule, overnight shifts reduced from 36 to 30 hours.

"That still seems like a lot of hours," I say, asking him if fatigue ever impairs his judgment.

"When I get tired," he says, "I get frustrated and I'm probably not as nice as I like to be. But I don't think the quality of my work suffers. I don't think I make mistakes."

Frank Luccia, who has two physician brothers, is married and in his late twenties. Though he is constantly in motion and hard to pin down, he says he agrees with Jim that life at this hospital is better than most. But he thinks the stress could be reduced more. "We would learn more if we had four or five patients," he says, rushing off somewhere, "instead of six, or eight, or nine."

Benjamin Frain, a twenty-four-year-old intern with dark good looks, a matinee idol's smile, and the intensity of an intellectual anxious to get his point across, is the team's major voice of dissension. He dismisses the residency system as "barbaric" and thinks it

---

*"Scut" refers to work that is menial or does not require a medical degree. This includes drawing blood, chasing down orders and X rays, scheduling tests, and transporting patients.

should be scrapped. "They are asking us to sacrifice our youth, our families, and our health," he says, "for a system that could be considerably more efficient and humane." Benjamin says he is switching to a psychiatry residency next year not only because the hours are better—psychiatrists typically are on call about once a week—but because he has a philosophical problem with spending so much time in the hospital. "I think a doctor needs to be well balanced," he says. "How can I be a good doctor if I don't know about life?"

Team Alpha's third and final intern, twenty-nine-year-old Gregory Kuhn, doesn't want to talk about residency reform or anything else this morning. Lean and tall like a basketball player, he has been awake and working at the hospital since seven yesterday morning. His eyes are glazed and puffy. He appears to be functioning all right, though his exhaustion has squeezed out any semblance of personality, curiosity, or politeness. Every movement and utterance is a chore. At one point he looks as if he might get sick, and sits down. Jim asks if he feels okay.

"Yeah," Gregory says, frowning. "I have that shitty-stomach-after-call feeling."

The two medical students on Team Alpha are in their late twenties. Both are on a medical research track, stretching their training out beyond the usual four years of medical school and the three to five years of residency to earn Ph.D.'s. Janice Walker, twenty-nine, has a Ph.D. in medical engineering. She is engaged to a chemistry professor in the Midwest, whom she hasn't seen "for way too long." A quiet, methodical woman, she is worried about how she can have children and finish the remaining seven years of her training. "It bothers my fiancé that I'm going to have no time to do outside things," she says. "He's finished his Ph.D. and wants to live a normal life."

Randolf Martin, also twenty-nine years old, is finishing a Ph.D. in medical anthropology, studying how doctors interact with each other and with patients. "The world of the doctor," he tells me, as if he is observing some exotic tribe on a lost island, "has a peculiar code of heroics, self-denial, and stress—it's a culture of stress."

■

After morning rounds, the team converges on the fourth floor's workstation—a study in drab beige hues, with several nondescript desks, a Formica counter, and telephones—to write up orders, scribble out progress notes, and confer with nurses. Jim tries to talk the radiology people into bringing their portable machine up to scan a woman he says should not be moved. "Rays," though, say they are too busy. They can't do it until tomorrow. Jim decides she needs a scan anyway and calls into the the hospital basement to ask for an orderly. He's told there are none available. "I'll end up carting her down to rays myself," he says, sounding frustrated, "or no one will."

I remind him that a few minutes earlier he was telling me the hospital holds his hand on this sort of scut.

"There's a shortage of orderlies and nurses," he says, shrugging. "That means we sometimes get stuck doing the scut. But the hospital is at least trying."

After a quick breakfast, the team settles down for attending rounds in the fourth floor conference room. Dr. George Bernard, a sixtyish infectious disease specialist, is this month's attending for Team Alpha, the physician ultimately responsible for the patients on the fourth floor. He listens while Frank and the interns present their twenty-two patients. Gregory starts with a cardiac patient, a fifty-year-old whose angina became unstable during the night. The shrill *beeeeeep!* of pagers frequently interrupts the meeting as team members pop up and down to answer calls. According to a study published in the *New England Journal of Medicine*, beepers interrupted residents surveyed up to twenty-five times in a single night. One resident told me she had developed a Pavlovian response to her pager. Every time the buzzer went off, she said, the noise made her nauseated, as if she wanted to vomit. She had to switch to a vibrating pager.

Looking more exhausted by the minute, Gregory presents a patient who came into the emergency room overnight with pneumonia and dizziness. Male. Seventy-five. Smoker for sixty years. Liver problems. "For a while he was going down fast," says Gregory, who adds he nearly panicked. "Just call me a chicken intern at three A.M.," he says. Dr. Bernard moves to the chalkboard to go over possible diagnoses. He has an easygoing, competent teaching style that leaves the team feeling at ease. Benjamin told me this is not always the case. "You get all kinds," he said later. "Some attendings find it a chore and leave us hanging, and then just show up to sign off on the notes."

"And what's the patient's mental status?" asks Dr. Bernard.

"Waning," says Gregory, who zones out for a moment as the team discusses a possible neurological disorder. Dr. Bernard asks Jim, as today's intern on call, to order a CT scan.*

"Whoa," says Gregory, breaking out of his lethargy. His speech is slow and slightly slurred. "Time out, I spaced out. I did a CT. There was nothing significant."

Moments later, with Gregory's portion of attending rounds over, he is asleep sitting in his chair. No one seems to notice. Afterward, I ask Jim if he thought Gregory sounded tired. "A little," he says, "but he did fine."

"But he forgot things. He was slurring words."

"He had a rough night," says Jim, "but he wasn't impaired."

■

Attending rounds last from ten to noon, with each patient offering a peculiar set of problems that have to be analyzed and acted on. I am astonished by the complexity of the cases, and the breadth of knowledge required to function in a ward where profound ethical and social dilemmas are daily fare. Does this woman have TB, or emphysema? What's her BUN, her creatinine, her sodium, her bicarb? What did the social worker say about Mrs. G.'s qualifying for a nursing home? Is that man HIV positive? Are we really going to patch that woman up just so she can go out and shoot up again? Is he too old for surgery—should we just let him die in peace? Toward the end, Jim presents Mary Allen. Frank asks if the family has okayed a DNR yet. No, answers Jim. "There's sort of a rift between the two daughters," he says, with one being "reasonable"—that is, she's going along with the doctors' recommendation to go DNR. "The other one," says Jim, "isn't very reasonable."

"I want you to call them," says Frank forcefully as the meeting breaks up, "and tell them things are irreversible." Jim goes to the phone and tries, but no one is home. He tells me he wishes he hadn't let things get this far, that he had taken the time to get the DNR earlier. "This lady is just really uncomfortable," he says worriedly.

Unable to reach Mary Allen's family, Jim decides he had better go to lunch while he can. We go out on the hospital lawn, where he sits

*Computerized Axial Tomography.

basking in the sunshine. "This is great," he says. "I never get outside anymore during daylight hours." But before he gets halfway through his chicken pita sandwich, he's beeped with his first admission of the day, a seventy-seven-year-old man with a heart valve that is severely narrowed, forcing his heart to work overtime, and depriving him of a steady supply of oxygenated blood. Several days earlier, cardiologists had performed a valvuloplasty, inserting a tiny balloon into his heart that's inflated to force open the valve. But it didn't work. In the busy E.R., curtained off from other patients, Jim does a quick physical and tries to convince the man to consider open heart surgery, an option he has so far refused.

I try to listen, but it's hard to hear—or, for that matter, to think. Overhead intercoms shout a steady babble of requests for this doctor or that emergency team. Monitors beep and hum, and busy people in scrubs and white coats bustle about. Shelves line the walls, brimming over with supplies. Trash bins and "medical refuse" canisters overflow onto the floor. Behind another curtain, only partially pulled, a man curses loudly, demanding morphine. He's young and high. A lab team arrives wearing heavy gloves and goggles, I assume as a precaution against HIV, though they may simply be loath to touch a man covered with what looks like vomit. One of the nurses threatens to call security if he doesn't shut up.

Jim's patient, a quiet, dignified old man, is obviously disturbed by the commotion. He's becoming disoriented. Jim seems oblivious to the fact he is asking an old man to make a difficult, possibly life-and-death decision in what must seem to him a madhouse. He mutters to me that the guy seems to be developing a mental status problem. The patient finally says he doesn't want surgery because he's "too old to get all cut up." Jim shakes his head as we walk away and says, "How unreasonable can you get?" I tell him that's the second time he's called a patient unreasonable because they did not agree with him. "Really?" he says. "I guess that's not a very good choice of words. It's just that patients and families sometimes lack the knowledge and the information to make good decisions. They become very emotional. In the old days, doctors just said, 'Here's what we're doing,' and patients said, 'Okay, whatever you say.' Now patients want to decide. I'm not sure if this is always the best way."

■

That afternoon Jim sees two patients in the hospital's outpatient clinic, joins Team Alpha for "ray rounds" to check X rays with a radiologist, and then tries to catch up on his "things to do" list, which runs several pages. At 4:15, Frank leads another blitzkrieg run through the patients with Jim, Benjamin, and the medical students. Gregory, who was supposed to go home at noon under the hospital's new policy of thirty-hour shifts, is still here; he will go home after rounds, finishing off a thirty-five-hour day. Frank Luccia, flipping through charts, groans when he sees that several orders have not been done—I.V.'s not started and tests not done. In a low, irritated mutter he tells me this is what runs a resident ragged. "So much slips between the cracks," he says, "and we're the fail-safe. This can really piss you off when you're up all night because you've been chasing down X rays."

Frank reminds Jim to call Mary Allen's family. "I'm guessing she'll die tonight," he says. Jim tries a number, but no one is home. We walk up to Mary's room on the sixth floor. She is wide awake, her frail gray body heaving. Jim orders an oxygen mask and the Ativan, then returns to the fourth floor to check other patients, write up the heart valve admission, and catch up on orders. He's beeped three times in rapid succession as we walk down the hall.

At 6:30, a nurse on the sixth floor pages Jim to tell him Mary Allen is trying to take off her mask and get out of bed. When we arrive, a nurse is holding her down. "She's surprisingly strong," says the nurse. Jim firmly pushes Mary down, shouting to her: "Why can't you leave that on for me?" Mary gives up and looks deeply into his eyes. "Help me," she moans, her chest heavy with fluid slowly squeezing the life out of her lungs. "I can't breathe."

At seven P.M., two of Mary's daughters show up on their own and Jim tells them their mother is dying. One of the daughters is still not sure about the DNR. "Can't the lungs be drained?" she asks. They go in to see their mother. When Mary sees them, she screams and tries to get up. The daughters cry and hug her as nurses bring in monitoring equipment and hook up more I.V.'s. The residents try putting in a stronger sedative. But Mary's veins are so emaciated they keep "blowing out." She is in obvious pain, her eyes wide with terror. Jim is so distraught he has let the situation come to this, that his patient is in pain because he didn't get the DNR, he steps into a supply room to compose himself. Later he told me he almost cried. His bloodshot eyes suggest he did.

A few minutes later, Frank is talking to the family in the hallway. "It's unlikely she'll turn around," he says calmly. "My advice to you is to make her comfortable," meaning they should go with the morphine. "If she were a family member of mine, I'd not want heroics."

When two of Mary's sisters arrive, the residents convince the daughters to go with the morphine and let their mother die. But now her paper-thin veins won't take the drip. Barely able to contain his frustration, Jim grabs a syringe and injects the morphine directly. But it is too late to ease Mary Allen's pain. She dies in agony a few minutes later, at eight-thirty-five P.M. But before this happens, Jim's beeper starts going crazy. Two more admissions are waiting for him in the emergency room. While he is gone, Mary Allen slips away. Later, when we return to her room so Jim can pronounce her dead, he tells me it was horrible, just horrible not to be there at the final moment. But he looks relieved, because her misery is finally over. In death, Mary Allen looks serene at last.

■

In the E.R., a Jordanian woman who has suffered a mild stroke is stable enough to be sent upstairs to a room for Jim to visit later. Stern's other admission is an eighty-seven-year-old former cantor who is blind; he has Alzheimer's and suffers from numerous chronic but stable conditions. He is here now because an E.R. resident thinks he has pneumonia. Randolf, the medical student, has joined us. He will write up and present the cantor on rounds the next morning.

As it turns out, the E.R. resident, his shift over after sixteen hours, went home before all the test results came back. Jim puts a question mark by the diagnosis of pneumonia. "I was afraid of this," he says. "They were in a shift change. I should have been here. Things didn't get done." Later, the tests will show that the E.R. resident, coming off a grueling all-night stint in the most hectic part of the hospital, and helping out Jim despite his own full load of patients, was wrong about the pneumonia. This wouldn't have mattered, except that he had already started the old man on a powerful antibiotic, thinking he had better do something before he left. "These are very strong drugs for an old man," says Jim. "They will wipe out his immune system for a while."

"Is he in danger?" I ask.

"Not really," he says, "but it's not good. He'll have to stay here a few days instead of going home."

I ask Jim how often this sort of thing happens, and he assures me that life-threatening errors are rare. "We have good backup," he says. "People are always watching us." He admits that minor things happen all the time, however. "An order isn't filled, or whatever, and a patient is uncomfortable."

"Like Mary Allen," I say.

"Yeah," says Jim. "Like Mary Allen."

Later, I asked Jim Stern's hospital for statistics on residents' errors. Not surprisingly, they said comprehensive records are not kept. I was assured by Jim's superiors that mistakes are infrequent. "Possibly a handful each year," said the chief of Jim's department. But even during my thirty-one hour stint following Jim Stern, I saw three situations that I would call errors; and were identified as such by Stern, or someone else present, or later when I reviewed the events of the day with Stern's chief resident. These included Mary Allen and the cantor who received antibiotics he didn't need. Another intern wrote an extra zero on a dosage order for a powerful narcotic, which was caught by a pharmacist. It was "a close one," said the resident.

At 9:50, Jim sends the Cantor upstairs and we grab a quick dinner of burned macaroni and cheese in a special night-call cafeteria for residents, an unappetizing place in the "bowels" of the hospital not far from where garbage is stored. Here Jim briefly sees his wife, an OB-GYN resident also on call that night. They talk as he tanks up on coffee and shovels food into his mouth. He gives her a quick kiss and we head back upstairs.

After briefly looking in on several patients and checking their charts, we visit the Jordanian woman admitted that afternoon. Jim tries to give her a physical and to take a history, but she speaks no English. Unable to ask her what is wrong, he decides he can't do anything but keep her stable until a translator can be found in the morning, even though she is obviously in pain. (A translator had been available earlier, but Jim was too busy.) After checking on another admission sent up from the E.R., a demented ninety-two-year-old man with a faulty heart valve, Jim sits down at the Team Alpha station to get caught up on his paperwork. His desk is piled high with charts, order slips, and lab results.

At 11:30 P.M., the pandemonium of the day and evening on the wards finally calms down as Jim Stern settles in at his station. Down the three hallways leading off from the station, someone has switched off every other bank of lights. Machines whir quietly and sometimes beep. Nurses checking patients occasionally pace up and down the halls. One of them wears hard heels that go clickity-clack, echoing in the night. Every few minutes, the ninety-two-year-old man cries out loudly for no apparent reason, sounding as if he's being tortured. Otherwise, an eerie quiet settles over the ward.

Jim begins writing up long, detailed descriptions of his patients, and what happened today, his pen making scratching noises on the charts as he records everything that happened that day—lab results, patient plans, and possible diagnoses. I notice he is writing in long-hand at a station that has no typewriters and only one computer, used almost exclusively for transmitting lab data. His work area is remarkably low tech in a hospital brimming with advanced medical equipment. Incredibly, the resident's phones are still rotary dial.

At four A.M., Jim sees that I'm struggling to stay awake and orders me to bed. He promises to wake me if anything happens. I gladly lie down on a bunk bed in Team Alpha's small on-call room behind the station. I'm awakened only once, when Jim goes to bed, fully clothed. I look at my watch. It's 6:30 A.M.

Fifty-five minutes later, Jim is up. It's 7:25, and he's got five minutes to splash water on his face before morning rounds. Outside the on-call room, the team is assembling for what will be a repeat of yesterday's morning—early rounds, placing orders with nurses, a quick breakfast, and attending rounds with Dr. Bernard. Today, however, it is Jim Stern who is exhausted and complaining of "that shitty-stomach-after-call feeling." Like Gregory the day before, he gives a competent presentation of his patients, though his answers are slow, with long pauses and occasional slurred speech. (I find myself unable to concentrate; my notes in my reporter's pad are noticeably sloppier and less coherent as I sip scalding hot coffee to keep from falling asleep. Another trick residents use is to suck on ice chips to stay awake.) Jim is far less patient and easygoing than the day before. I recall that yesterday he told me fatigue did not affect him, and I realize he probably needs to believe this. When Dr. Bernard moves on to hear Benjamin's presentations, Jim nods off. A few minutes later, I join him, still sitting up in my chair at the conference table.

■

For the rest of the morning Jim's patients remained stable, which meant he would get to go home close to on time, at noon. This does not always happen. All it takes is for one patient to develop a problem anytime before he leaves, and he has to stay, sometimes for hours. Jim told me he had never stayed post call past supper time, though other residents said they had slugged it out as late as ten or eleven P.M. This put them over the top of forty hours in a single shift.

At 1:45 P.M., after rounds with Dr. Bernard, Jim Stern finally signs over his patients to Benjamin, who is on call today. He then takes off his sweat-stained scrub shirt and washes his upper body in the call room while I jot down a quick breakdown of what he did over the past thirty-one hours:

> With patients: 4 hours
> Education/rounds: 5 hours
> Writing notes/orders/phone: 15.5 hours
> "Scut" work: 4 hours
> Sleep: 55 minutes
> Eating/personal: 1.5 hours

Jim is taken aback by how little time he spent with patients, and admits this part of his training is seriously lacking. He also is surprised by the nearly sixteen hours of paperwork. I ask him if he has ever considered using a computer. He says he would love to, but he doesn't have the time to learn how to use one. Nor does the hospital have any plans to teach him, he said.

At 1:53 P.M., almost thirty-one hours after he arrived at the hospital, Jim finally leaves. He crosses the street and meets his wife in a pub for a beer and lunch. They tell me when I join them that today is Jim's twenty-ninth birthday. I ask what he's going to do to celebrate, and he and his wife, both too exhausted even to eat, answer wearily: "We're going home to sleep."

CHAPTER I

Means to an End?

*So act as to treat humanity, whether in thine own person
or in that of any other, in every case as an end withal,
never as means only . . .*

Immanuel Kant

Three years after Mary Allen died, Jim Stern's skin is no longer the color of chalk. He's lost the swollen circles under his eyes, put on weight, and trimmed his dark hair back to an athletic-looking burr cut. But the most striking change in Jim Stern is his attitude. Now finished with his residency, and nine months into a three-year cardiology fellowship, he strides down the hall of his hospital with an authority that is astonishing compared to the overwhelmed, pushed-to-the-edge intern driven to despair because he allowed an old woman to suffer needlessly.

"You gain a lot of confidence as you become more senior in the system, as you learn more," says Stern, walking into a small office in his hospital's basement, which he shares with a half-dozen other fellows. He grabs a muffin and a large bag of pretzels—"dinner," he says—and leads me into one of the seemingly endless, nondescript conference rooms in his hospital. Once there, he begins devouring the pretzels methodically, as if he's timing the pickup, delivery, and chewing of each and every one.

I ask Stern what he remembers about that night three years ago. He surprises me by saying it was a slow one. He apologizes for what he says must have been "a boring experience, since nothing happened." Then I remind him of Mary Allen—and the cantor, and all the rest. As I speak, and he looks over my notes from that night, the progression of pretzels slows and then stops. "I had completely forgotten about all of this," he says, the color in his face turning a shade paler. "That was a nightmare night. How could I have forgotten it?" He shakes his head. "I guess it's true what they say about forgetting the bad and remembering the good. But it's all coming back now."

He talks about Mary Allen, saying: "It's my recollection that the question was whether or not to give a drug we knew had a good chance of hastening her demise, even though it would make her comfortable. And there was a family disagreement about that. And we waited too long, and then we couldn't get the I.V. in, which was extremely frustrating." He says he remembers feeling overwhelmed, angry—and, recalling the supply room scene, helpless. "I was way behind," he says, "and then I got into a situation where I was not confident with my medical, legal, or ethical standing, and a woman suffered."

As Stern spoke, for just an instant I saw a look of tentativeness flash across his face, that sense of not quite knowing what to do or say that at times had been so disconcerting three years earlier. "That should not have happened," he said, staring at the pretzel he had been holding in his hand. "It wouldn't happen to me today. I would be more aggressive. I would sit the family down and make them make the decision about the DNR. I would probably go ahead and give the patient the morphine, because now I know that is the right thing to do."

■

The agony of Mary Allen is hardly a sensational story in these tabloid times. No one was killed or maimed, and there were no horrific or obvious errors that radically changed her condition for the worse. As Jim Stern rightly pointed out, Mary Allen was dying anyway, though he admits that he contributed to her passing away in less than ideal circumstances. Stern is also right in saying that he's far less likely to make the same mistake today. But he doesn't acknowledge, or perhaps realize what this means, that part of his confidence comes from the horror he felt for his part in causing an old woman to feel pain as she choked and gasped for air, and the terror of her own death rose up in her eyes.

The case of Mary Allen—and others like it—raises a crucial question about means justifying ends; about whether it's acceptable to allow even a single old woman to suffer so that a young physician can learn a valuable lesson. In *The Brothers Karamazov*, Fyodor Mikhailovich Dostoyevsky poses the same dilemma when Ivan Karamazov asks his brother Alyosha if he would be willing to build a society "with the aim of making men happy in the end, of giving them peace and contentment at last" if the price was "to torture to death only one tiny creature . . . and to found the edifice on her unavenged tears—would you consent to be the architect on those conditions? Tell me and do not lie!"

Few queries are more critical to understanding how raw medical recruits are shaped into healers—and why there exists such a powerful tension in medicine between its ideals, and a sometimes less than perfect reality.

Which brings us to a question we might as well ask straight away: Do residents hurt people? Do they occasionally kill them? Is it dangerous to be a patient in a teaching hospital?

For some physicians, raised in a culture where perfection (thankfully) is a virtual religion, and mistakes are viewed as rare aberrations, to even suggest such a thing is an ugly, insulting accusation. "It almost never happens," said a chief of general medicine at a well-known hospital, who blamed the media for sensationalizing a few tragic incidents. "This is a great, great disservice to the public, to residents, and to medicine," he said, looking me square in the eyes.

With equal passion, other physicians insist mistakes happen far too often. "Residents do kill people," an attending and educator in New York City told me, adding that inexperience, lack of supervision, and overwork can be a lethal combination. "Do you want me to give you an example from last week," he asked, his face turning red with indignation, "or the week before?"

■

If this were a book about airplane crashes, train derailments, industrial fatalities, mine shaft collapses, or the accidental venting of radioactive gas, I could list here with some precision how many persons are killed or injured who shouldn't be. For most cases, I could tell you whether or not human error or incompetence was to blame. Medicine, however, collects but little meaningful data on physician (or resident) error. In a way this is understandable, given the earth-scorching, no-holds-barred warfare that currently passes for law between plaintiffs' lawyers and physicians. Doctors also have been naturally loath over the years to make public their own mistakes, preferring either to ignore them or to deal with them internally. The public, by the way, has not complained about this until recently.

Another problem is the sheer complexity of disease, and identifying what actually caused a death or an unexpected outcome. Most cases are simply not as clear-cut as, say, the cause of death when a Boeing 747 falls out of the sky in a ball of flames. Did the patient die of bacterial infection, liver disease, renal failure, or a combination of all three? Did it matter that the intern waited a few hours longer than he should have to order antibiotics for a bacterial infection that might have killed the patient anyway? Could the PGY2 have saved the woman whose heart stopped and could not be restarted, if she had sent her more quickly to intensive care?

Cadavers carry no black box to explain what happened in the final days and hours of life—or who, if anyone, was at fault. Nor are organs and blood vessels created according to strict specifications, as are jet engines, wings, hydraulic systems, flaps, and landing gears. And as often as not, autopsies, when performed at all, are inconclusive while causation gets lost in the intricacies and complexities of physiology, disease, and treatment.

It can be equally difficult to decide what, exactly, *is* a mistake, beyond the obvious cases of amputating the wrong leg or punching a hole in a healthy intestine during an appendectomy. Is it a mistake if a surgeon takes a risk and fails to save someone dying from a life-threatening gunshot wound? Was it truly an error for Jim Stern to make the decision to let a terminal patient die, and then fail to get the family's consent to relieve the resulting pain and emotional distress?

All of this has relegated the issue to a kind of limbo between screaming headlines and anecdotes whispered in hospital corridors, told as believe-it-or-not tales about someone's sister or cousin who erroneously had their gallbladder removed, or nearly died when a drug order got mixed up.

Into this void comes a handful of physician-researchers who have begun to study the question of medical error. These include Dr. Lucian Leape, a tall, lanky, deep-voiced pediatric surgeon, sixty-four years old. Eight years ago he put down his scalpel and began writing seminal studies on medical outcomes at RAND and Harvard's School of Public Health. He also began asking serious questions about what role physician errors play when outcomes turn sour. Declaring that "mistakes are inevitable" in medicine, as they are elsewhere, Leape caused something of a sensation at Christmas time in 1994 when he estimated that 180,000 Americans die each year in part from *iatrogenic* injuries (those caused by the actions or attitude of physicians, or from treatment received as a patient in a hospital). Leape claimed that "most iatrogenic injuries are due to errors and are, therefore, potentially preventable," with proper safeguards—such as having correct drug dosages easily accessible on computers, and using appropriate training systems for residents and nurses. Writing in the high-profile *Journal of the American Medical Association* (*JAMA*), Leape based his conclusions on an extensive survey of available research on medical mistakes, including data on over 30,000 cases in New York state that he and a team of Harvard outcomes experts studied in 1991.

If Leape and his colleagues are right, then dozens of Americans are dying every day in part from iatrogenic injuries—"the equivalent of three jumbo-jet crashes every two days," says Leape.

In a field nearly bereft of serious research, the few studies on hand back up Lucian Leape's estimates. One recent survey of obtainable data concludes that one percent of all hospital patients "suffer harm because of substandard medical care." Of these, about 84,000 die, says the report, and 20,000 suffer permanent disability.

Another source of information on general medical errors is collected by a handful of states that require hospitals to report adverse events, particularly when errors cause injury or death. One of these is New York, which each year investigates thousands of cases reported to them by hospitals—which by law must inform the state of any untoward incident. According to the last year when data was published,* New York's 232 hospitals tallied 10,603 adverse events—equal to four per 1,000 patients discharged, with 464 of these resulting in death. Extrapolated out to the nation as a whole, these numbers equal more than 45,000 deaths each year because of medical errors. This is less than Leape's figure, though even this lower estimate is far higher than is tolerated in other industries where lives are at stake. For instance, in 1992, 33 people died in commercial airline crashes, and 40,000 died in motor vehicle accidents.

---

*Because of statewide budget cuts in New York, the state's department of health has not published data on reported incidents since 1989, though it continues to collect it.

■

Little of the available research focuses specifically on mistakes made by residents, though Leape and other experts say that the potential for errors is high among neophyte physicians, particularly interns and junior residents. This belief is supported by a scattering of studies that touch on resident mistakes, an area that has been virtually ignored as a topic for serious, systematic examination. Findings include:

- In New York, researchers discovered that academic teaching hospitals experienced a significantly higher rate of adverse events (4.1 percent of all cases studied) than nonteaching hospitals (2.3 percent), and those with limited teaching programs (3.4 percent).
- In JAMA, researchers reported that 45 percent of residents surveyed reported making a mistake, with 90 percent of these errors resulting in serious adverse outcomes for patients—including 31 percent who died. Only half the residents discussed their error with an attending physician; less than one in four told the patient or family.
- In Albany, New York, researchers at the Albany Medical Center Hospital singled out interns as being the worst offenders in errors involving prescribed drugs, with a rate of 4.25 mistakes for every 1,000 drug orders placed—compared to 3.3 per 1,000 for attendings. Over half of all errors in the study were "significant," resulting in some harm to patients, with 35 percent ranked as "severe," "serious," or "fatal."
- In a confidential survey of house staff errors in a respected East Coast hospital, researchers found that four out of five residents committed one or two errors in a single month. One-fifth said they made three to five mistakes. In close to half the cases, the patients reportedly experienced minor discomfort or inconvenience; 9 percent suffered minor complications and 3 percent major complications.

Another source for information comes from the incident reports in New York, though the state's department of health does not cull out incidents specifically caused by residents. In 1992, however, *New York Times* reporter Lisa Belkin, after spending several weeks perusing thousands of pages of state medical documents, concluded in a March 31 article that "One category of staff member receives a large percentage of the criticism in the incident reports—medical residents. . . . the questionable actions or lack of supervision of medical residents were cited as causes in a large number of the incidents investigated by the state." Belkin cited the following cases:

- At Beth Israel in New York City, a resident tried several times to insert a catheter into a patient's jugular vein, eventually puncturing the carotid artery, the major vessel supplying blood to the brain. Only after extensive bleeding had occurred did the resident call in a superior, but it was too late to save the patient. After the patient died, doctors found on autopsy two large holes in the artery. A hospital spokesperson said this was a common complication when inserting this type of catheter. "Most of the time it takes care of itself," he told Belkin.
- At Bronx Municipal Hospital, an anesthesiology resident mistakenly switched the inhalation and exhalation hoses on a ventilator during a hernia operation. Deprived of oxygen, the patient suffered cardiac arrest, and died six days later.
- At King's County Medical Center, a resident in the busy emergency room failed to notice a stab wound in the back of a young Hasidic scholar and left him sitting in the waiting room for hours, the first in a series of errors that also involved attendings and nurses. A few hours later, the patient died.

■

This admittedly sketchy data is supported by my own observations. Almost every time I followed a resident, I saw or heard about at least one mistake, most of them confirmed by the resident involved or someone familiar with the situation. These ranged from obvious diagnoses missed, which caused patients either discomfort or an extra day or two in the hospital, to lines and tubes being inserted incorrectly. During one bungled attempt to place a central venous line, performed by an unsupervised resident still trying to master this procedure, he hit the carotid artery and sent a geyser of blood spraying my way. It splattered my shirt and reporter's notebook.

I saw dosages mixed up, drugs given that shouldn't have been, orders forgotten, and procedures put off—sometimes for days because the resident forgot, was too busy, or simply had no idea what he or she was doing. In one hospital, I asked a surgical resident if it was dangerous to give residents so much responsibility. He told me about a drunk he saw come into his hospital's emergency room two weeks earlier. The man was cursing everyone and had to be restrained by security. A frustrated resident ordered him sedated but gave him too much of a potent narcotic. "This should not have happened," said the surgical resident. "He could have stopped breathing. Is that dangerous enough?"

Another resident in general medicine told me about a nephrology (kidney) patient who developed congestive heart failure because he gave the patient too much intravenous fluid too fast. Overwhelmed by a ward full of patients just a few weeks after graduating from medical school, he says he forgot to order the fluids reduced at the proper time. The patient died, he said, because of a heart attack brought on in part by the high pressure of too much liquid in his system. "This still keeps me up at night," he said. "It was horrible."

A first-year surgical resident in New England told me about a man coming into his hospital's busy urban emergency room after a barroom brawl. Though he was injured enough to rank as a major trauma, the residents did not run all the usual tests to determine if there was internal bleeding, thinking he was basically okay. "As he started to sober up, he started complaining, 'Oh, my stomach is killing me,' " one of the residents on call that night recalled, "and he started screaming more and more. We did a CT scan on him. He had a huge laceration in his spleen. He went right to the O.R. to get his spleen removed. He did fine. But if he hadn't complained, we would have let him go home and bleed to death."

An anesthesiology fellow who recently completed her four-year residency grew pensive and uncharacteristically sad after relating story after story of resident mistakes in her hospital. She said she "wanted to be upbeat" about her experience, because she loved being a doctor, liked her hospital, and respected most of her colleagues. "But I have to be honest," she said. "These things happen far too often that are not caught."

■

This brings us back to Mary Allen—and Dostoyevsky—and what is perhaps the most prickly question of all: do residents *need* to inconvenience, hurt, and even occasionally kill patients in order to learn?

Historically, when the modern residency system was developed late in the last century and early in this one, the answers were more clear. This is because few in medicine really questioned the basic premise of the teaching hospital; these were places where physicians learned and perfected their craft on a population predominately poor and often destitute (or exotic or seemingly incurable), who typically had no choice but to trade the uncertainty of being handled by trainees and other physicians for free or almost free care. This was long before Medicare, Medicaid, employer-sponsored Health Maintenance Organizations, and COBRA,* when doctors treated wealthier patients at home, in sanitariums, in private offices, and in early prototypes of what we now call community hospitals.

This is not to say that poor patients were left at the mercy of coldhearted physician–scientists to do as they pleased. In fact, hospital boards (some of which included doctors) frequently admonished physicians to place a higher priority on the well-being of the patient, however destitute, than on teaching and research—a situation that created considerable tension in the nineteenth and early twentieth centuries, and to a lesser extent up until the present. Nor does it mean that physicians, individually or as a group, were more callous or less committed to a patient's well-being before 1965, when Congress enacted Medicaid and Medicare. One only need look around a hospital room, or O.R., to see that physicians collectively over the past century have contributed mightily to improving everyone's health. It can even be argued, as crass as it may sound, that without the charity patients set aside as test subjects for doctor trainees, physicians would not have become as proficient as they did in the early stages of modern medicine.

Times have changed, however. "When I was finishing medical

*Consolidated Omnibus Budget Reconciliation Act, a 1985 act of Congress that restructured federal expenditures for and regulation of health care in the United States.

school," says Dr. Bertrand Bell, professor of medicine at the Albert Einstein College of Medicine, who trained in the mid-fifties, "the place everybody wanted to train was the public hospital. Why? It was unsupervised, and the trade-off was you take care of the poor in exchange for learning. In my day, everything was noblesse oblige. We're going to take care of these people and learn from them, and if they did it right, the patients did all right. And if they died, well, that was too bad, but that's the risk they took coming to the charity wards.

"History has moved forward since I trained," notes Bell, a small, wiry primary care specialist and vociferous critic of the modern residency system. In 1987, he chaired the state commission that suggested New York regulate resident work hours and increase supervision—rules the state adopted in 1989. "Today most patients in teaching hospitals are paying customers," he says. "Yet here we are, forty years down the pike, and they're doing the same thing at most hospitals. Treating paying customers like they're indigents who supposedly won't care if you let loose undersupervised, inexperienced doctors to work on them."

Edmund Pellegrino, a highly respected internist and former president of Yale/New Haven Medical Center, who now heads the Center for Clinical Bioethics at Georgetown University, also has little patience for medical educators who believe that "the university hospital is all a laboratory. But what do patients come in here for?" asks Pellegrino. "To be cared for. Not for students primarily to be taught, or for research."

Bell and other reformers contend that a fundamental crisis exists in many teaching hospitals because they haven't kept up with a public that now refuses to go along with the old trade-off—not only because they are paying customers, but because the ethics of patients' participation in their own care has shifted from the doctor-knows-best model to what medical ethicists call "patient autonomy." Competition is also straining the old system of training, as viable alternatives have sprung up to compete with academic hospitals. "There are good hospitals now in suburbia run by experienced attendings and nurses," says Bell, "so people don't always want to come in anymore to a teaching hospital. Why should they, if we aren't treating them right?"

■

In one of the larger teaching hospitals in America, a sprawling complex of buildings ranging from a century old to brand new, an attending-educator clips an X ray onto a light board. Some forty physicians, including twenty-six residents, look on, a standing-room-only crowd in the internal medicine department's library. Surrounded by shelves of heavy textbooks and journals, and by composite photos of every medical residency class in the hospital's history hanging on the walls, the attending begins to speak. "This case concerns a fifty-two-year-old male picked up by an EMS* at a dialysis center," he says. "The man complained of pain in his chest, spreading laterally into his back. He also said he had been vomiting blood." A thin, balding man dressed in an expensive shirt and tie under his lab coat, the attending delivers a concise history of the patient whose fuzzy organs and rib cage appear in the X ray. Speaking in a near-monotone, he recounts the patient's vital signs, "a blood pressure of 210/110; heart rate 92; respiration 30 . . ."

This gathering is called a Mortality and Morbidity Conference—an "M & M" in physician parlance. Long a tradition in teaching hospitals, its purpose is to see if a predicted outcome actually occurred, and to analyze what happened if things went wrong, particularly if someone made an obvious error. In this case, a fifty-two-year-old man with a failing liver, bad kidneys, and a weak heart had died after repeated vomiting tore a hole in his esophagus. Apparently this was caused or greatly aggravated by the fact the resident team (and several attendings) had overlooked a serious internal bleed, until it was too late.

As the attending and others slowly unravel the events leading to the man's death, everyone in the room avoids glancing at an intern sitting next to a shelf of medical texts. He is in his late twenties, with a skinny frame and a mustache composed of just a few long black hairs. "He's the one who first missed the diagnosis," whispers the resident I am with, "because he didn't get a critical part of the patient's history. He wasn't the only one to miss it, but it was his patient who died."

A few minutes later, the intern himself is asked to stand and offer his version of what went wrong. Stoically, he explains the crux of his team's error—that it was two days before they discovered that the man had been vomiting "chocolate-covered material" at home, a telltale sign of internal bleeding. Had the doctors known this, the attending notes somberly, they would have treated him

*Emergency Medical Service, i.e., an ambulance service.

differently—and might have saved his life. Instead, the man deteriorated rapidly and coded three times, dying three days after his admission.

This prompts an older physician in a crisp white coat to raise his hand and offer the first comment not delivered in a bland, scientific tone. "But why didn't you take a good history in the first place?" he asks angrily. "The patient was alert. His wife was there. This is unbelievable!"

The intern blanches, and everyone in the room seems to hold their breath, knowing that in years past an M & M was as often as not a grilling session to chew out an erring resident. When no one else joins in the older doctor's ire, the meeting continues as before, the speech returning to a neutral, nuts-and-bolts discussion, as if this were a meeting of automobile mechanics pondering a recalcitrant carburetor.

■

In virtually all teaching hospitals, M & Ms are the only official, routine acknowledgment of errors by physicians. They are almost always held in private, with only residents and attendings present, and no real records kept. Most hospitals also have "risk assessment" and "quality of care" committees to handle serious errors, particularly those involving potential lawsuits, though these vary greatly from hospital to hospital. Some merely set vague guidelines for patient care; others maintain strict rules and rigorously investigate aberrations in patient safety and care, being aggressively proactive on their patients' behalf. Occasionally a hospital's ethics panel might step in, deliberating about what a patient and family have a right to know about mistakes, and about legal ramifications when cases go wrong.

Yet no ethics panel of which I am aware has ever discussed the larger issue of what mistakes, if any, are necessary for training physicians, and the morality of a system that seems to utilize errors as a training tool. "The profession of medicine has not approached this issue with the reverence it seems to deserve," commented researchers in Oregon, writing a paper on physician error.

Moreover, most M & Ms, patient care committees, and ethics panels consider only a small fraction of cases where transgressions occur. Indeed, if Leape and others are correct in their numbers, then the vast majority of iatrogenic incidents are never aired or talked about, even behind the closed doors of an M & M. This suggests that inasmuch as educators are aware that errors occur, at least some are officially ignored, apparently tolerated as a rueful but necessary price for training young physicians.

This is the central premise in a book published in 1979 by sociologist Charles L. Bosk. After spending eighteen months following surgeons around in the anonymous "Pacific Hospital," he assembled in his text a rich, if chilling, portrait of a culture that has come to believe that mistakes are regrettable but remain a necessary component of training. Titled *Forgive and Remember: Managing Medical Failure*, Bosk's book stands virtually alone among the sparse offerings on this subject in frankly admitting that errors happen on a routine basis—an assessment in which the author's surgeon-subjects tacitly concur. In fact, Bosk defines the role of the surgeon-educator as one who attempts to "control his subordinates' performance and make sure that errors are corrected and not repeated." At the same time, "he must allow his subordinates room to make errors or they will never learn the judgments and techniques necessary to perform properly."

Bosk fills his book with a sobering progression of quotes and stories from Pacific Hospital surgeons describing their mistakes—and how they or their trainees learned from them. He also goes to some pains to let the surgeons give their rationale. For instance, he quotes a PGY1 as insisting: "Of course I worry about making a mistake and it really being disastrous for a patient. But really the crime is not making a mistake; everybody is going to make mistakes. The crime is not learning from your errors. . . . For example, once I can remember sending home a young girl who came into the emergency room at four in the morning and who had abdominal pains and couldn't urinate. I was lucky somebody read over what I had done the next day and said: 'Good God, get her back right away—she has appendicitis.' So they brought her back and operated that afternoon and she did have appendicitis. That was a case of me not knowing enough and making the wrong decision, but nothing like that will ever happen again. I learned from it."

One wonders if the surgeons informed the family that a first-year doctor had fumbled, and that his inexperience had not only caused their little girl to suffer needlessly, but also exposed her to a risk of severe infection, or worse, had the appendix ruptured. How would they have reacted to reading Bosk's quote, and the notion that their daughter's close call was simply one of those errors educators expect when training young physicians?

■

Critics such as Lucian Leape and Bertrand Bell describe the current system of M & M critiques, near misses, unreported incidents, and informal dress-downs as a weak response that is at best outdated, at worst a potential hazard for patients. "Patients want to, and deserve to know when mistakes happen," says Bell. "They deserve to not be used as guinea pigs to train young doctors."

Lucian Leape is less caustic than Bell in his criticism. "For humans, the usual way we learn is by making mistakes," he contends, "and this is inevitable, and not necessarily bad—unless it hurts people." What concerns him is that physicians and hospitals do cause harm on occasion, yet they continue to act as though nothing can be done when, in fact, there are ways to prevent many common mistakes. He and a small band of like-minded physicians have proposed a number of measures to counter what he calls "adverse outcomes," such as using computers to assist doctors in having on hand critical information about patient histories, allergies, information on drugs, and allowable drug dosages.

"Most doctors practice the way doctors practiced in 1950," says Leape. "Fundamentally, we still operate on the principle that the physician should bring to the patient an immense amount of knowledge, and hopefully some wisdom, all of which he carries around in his head. We tend to rely too much on remembering everything, which is impossible given all we need to know."

According to Leape, writing in his 1994 *JAMA* article, the explanation for medicine's reluctance to confront and deal with errors starts with the way physicians are educated, and with a "paradox" that exists when "the standard of medical practice is perfection," while at the same time "all physicians recognize that mistakes are inevitable."

After reading this, I called Leape and asked him about the morality of this situation, how physicians charged first and foremost with doing no harm to patients could allow this paradox to continue.

First, he said, errors are random and rare enough that individual physicians are unaware of the collective scope of the problem. He also mentioned fear—of litigation, of what colleagues would think, of patients and families feeling as if their trust had been violated, of admitting to themselves they had made a mistake.

I asked Leape if it is ethical for the profession to downplay errors once the scope of the problem becomes clear. "I think we are kind of immune to them," said Leape. "We know that most of the time we don't make mistakes. I think most doctors look at them and say, well, you are going to have a certain amount and there's nothing you can do about it. Certainly they don't think about it in moral terms." This is because medical errors occur not in fiery, highly public crashes, but one by one in thousands of hospitals, offices, and clinics.

This reminds me of a director of a surgical residency program who assured me that residents make only "a few" mistakes in the course of their education. "Most might make one mistake a year that causes problems for a patient," he said. Possibly he had not stopped to figure the math, or to realize that if every resident and fellow errs once each year, this would equal 100,000 mistakes, a rate of 274 a day across the country.

"If doctors felt more of a moral obligation, knowing these things are preventable," said Leape, "then they would be more inclined to do the types of things it takes to make it happen."

■

Leape's sobering observations led me to seek out one cool autumn day in Baltimore the philosopher Stephen Vicchio, who teaches ethics at Johns Hopkins Medical School. I asked if it was fundamentally ethical to allow inexperienced residents to learn the art of medicine on real people, asking him to consider what would happen if the typical residency program in the United States was a new drug, never before tried on humans, one that researchers wanted permission to test from the Federal Drug Administration. Would it pass muster, or would it be rejected as too experimental and dangerous?

Vicchio, a big man whose linebacker's build belies gentle eyes and a quiet humor, guessed the latter. "It would be hard to defend this system purely in terms of patient safety," he said, though he immediately shot back with the crucial problem in my scenario: without hands-on training, we would have no experienced doctors.

This led him to pose a question of his own—which he then answered. "If it's a choice between having no physicians, where millions suffer, and hurting a few patients, which is worse? I'll tell you," he said. "First we have to ask if the mistakes were avoidable. If they were, and flaws in the system, or incompetence, or fatigue, or lack of supervision is involved, then hurting even one patient is wrong. Does that *still* override the imperative to train new doctors? I would say no, not if it's within our power to save these patients."

But this is the rub: what is within our power to thwart, and what is not? And if what Leape reports is true, why are physicians not rushing to scrutinize the cause and prevention of conditions that might save thousands or tens of thousands of lives—particularly as it applies to educating their own young?

■

Having suggested that residents make mistakes, I want to emphasize an important caveat—that the vast majority of the time, residents do *not* make errors. At times, it's exhilarating to watch young physicians learning their craft, and facing up to a world of death and dying that most of us would flee, particularly in an age when HIV, widespread drug abuse, child poverty, and teenage suicides are daily fare in most teaching hospitals. One can feel the learning curve surge upward as residents move from fumbling interns in their first weeks to competent physicians in the course of three to five years.

Yet the question remains: do patients (and residents) suffer undue harm from the current system? And what is it about this system that allows neophyte physicians to sometimes flounder about, inserting arterial lines without adequate training, dispensing drugs without really knowing proper doses, and running about trying to figure out what to do about a DNR order and a morphine injection when a patient is in agony?

CHAPTER 2

The Plunge-in Method

---

*It is clear . . . that a selective and varying, not an encyclo-
pedic or uniform, a lightly laden, not a too crowded curriculum offers the best opportunity for the training
requisite to mastery and growth.*

Abraham Flexner, M.D., 1925*

As best we can tell," says the rail-thin EMT with the Wyatt
Earp mustache, "three were in the pickup. Four were in the
van." He talks hurriedly, explaining details of a two-car, seven-per-
son crash to Claude Kelly, a PGY1 on his second night ever as an
intern. A quiet, exhausted twenty-seven-year-old with round
cheeks and green eyes, Kelly at 2:30 A.M. has been covering surgical
trauma in this busy emergency room for 17 1/2 hours—since seven
the previous morning. "Looked like the pickup spun the van
around. Guy driving the pickup was drunk. Blew through a stop
sign or something. He must have been cruising. Put one guy
through the windshield of the van. He went fifteen feet. Everybody
else was bloody and screaming. One was bleeding to death, I
thought. We got to her fast as we could. The truck went another
block from the force. Its windshield was a block away. The driver of
the pickup wasn't talking. I couldn't get him out of the truck. I had
to wait for special jaws to get there and open up the doors."

As he speaks, nurses and techs grab packets of I.V. solutions,
drugs, tubes, syringes, bandage kits, and sponges from open bins
attached to walls, painted red and blue. Monitors beep and click.
"Rays!" bellows a radiology tech, aiming a portable x-ray machine
at the van driver's chest—the one thrown fifteen feet. He moans in
pain, his head and upper body covered with blood. Everyone stands

*In 1910, Flexner wrote a critique of American medical schools, accusing some of them, among
other things, of failing to impart a vigorous scientific regimen, or a standard clinical experience. By
1925, Flexner was lamenting an overemphasis on rigid dogma at the expense of humanism in medical training.

clear as the x-ray device hums and clicks. Then they rush back into the garage-sized space, Trauma Room 3. EMTs wheel other crash victims into Trauma 1, Trauma 2, and Trauma 4.

In Trauma 3, Kelly's supervisor, the physician in charge of these four rooms, shouts orders to nurses and orderlies. "Okay, Mike," he yells at the driver of the van, who is groggy but awake, "we have to put a tube down your nose. Hold his head down," he tells an orderly the size of Arnold Schwarzenegger, and an equally formidable nurse, her girth being close to her height. "Hold his arms down to put the tube down. Swallow, Mike. Swallow."

I'll call this physician Bill Kidd, M.D. Cocky, confident, and as revved up as a bronco rider, he told me earlier, with an ironic laugh tempered by a boyish grin, that trauma was "the bad boy team, the guys who have to do it all." At first, I was put off by Kidd's bravado. But after awhile I warmed up to him, partly because he often interjected deprecating comments suggesting he's not such a "bad boy" after all. Later that night, glancing at the calmer, less explosive Claude Kelly, he said: "Claude's cool. Very cool. I've got to be more like Claude. You really have to be kind of hyper about all these things that might go wrong. But I need to do it calmly. I gotta remember that."

Like Kelly, Kidd is brand new at his job as teacher-supervisor. Neither an attending nor even a senior resident, he has just started his third year in surgery. This means he has only two years' experience behind him in a five-year program. For the moment, these two young doctors comprise the entire surgical trauma team covering the E.R.

Theoretically, they have backup—an emergency medicine attending and other residents in the main E.R., down the hall from trauma; a fifth-year chief resident, overseeing eight to ten interns and junior residents on call that night throughout the hospital; another PGY3 in the Surgical Intensive Care Unit (SICU); and surgical fellows in orthopedics and cardiothoracic surgery. Kidd and Kelly could also call the attending assigned that night to cover trauma, who was home in bed. When I asked Kidd about this, he laughed, saying no one ever bothered an attending at home unless it was an emergency requiring immediate surgery, which the attending was required to either perform himself, or to supervise in person. "Do I have a problem with calling the attending at 3 A.M. with just any old question?" Asks Kidd. "Yes."

"Why?"

"Because we're expected to do things on our own."

Kidd and Kelly tell me that most nights, the hospital's backup system works well enough. By "works" they mean that one or more E.R. attendings is usually available to help out, though Kidd says they are not qualified to handle level-one surgical trauma. During another evening I was in the E.R., a fifth-year surgical chief once poked his head into the trauma bay, but he stayed only briefly to check on a patient before heading into the O.R. for the rest of the night.

I later asked one of the veteran trauma nurses how often the system broke down. "There are ups and downs," she said. "There are a lot of times they are left trying to do too much. These are the new ones who are trying to learn the system. The ones that have been around awhile are generally very good."

Tonight, the system seems to be strained to the breaking point. It is a sweltering Saturday night in July—"a party hearty weekend," said one of the EMTs, rushing out to take another call. Swamped with cases at 2:30 A.M., a half-hour after bars close in this city, the hospital's immediate, in-house backup is too busy to help Kidd and Kelly. This leaves them on their own, a situation Kidd says he relishes. "We can handle it," he tells me. "We're trauma." He flashes his ironic grin. "Remember? We're the bad boys." He straps on an apron and a clear plastic shield to cover his face and eyes before going to work. He hands me another shield and orders me to slip it on, to guard against HIV or hepatitis-tainted blood splashing into my eyes.

With the trauma bays all full, and more patients waiting, the formidable-looking nurse suggests to Kidd he call in backup. He doesn't respond. A seven-year veteran of the trauma rooms, she turns to me with a shrug as she rummages through a bin, looking for sutures. "He really should call someone," she says. I ask if she would call in help if Kidd didn't. "That's not the way it works. That's not really done."

Across the room, Kidd knots up his thin, angular face, poised to jab a quarter-inch-thick clear plastic tube into the van driver's left nostril and down his esophagus. Called a nasogastric tube, or NG, it's used to suction out fluid from the stomach to check for internal bleeding. It takes a practiced hand to slip in the tube without tearing tissue in the nose or throat. "We can't give him a painkiller because that would mess up his neuro exam," says Kelly, referring to the fact that neurologists prefer to have their patients undrugged so they can accurately assess their mental status after being injured.

"*Arrrgghhhhh*," screams an obviously drunk and dazed Mike as Kidd bears down. "Come on, I'm dying."

"No, you're not dying," says Kidd.

"Let me out! *Arrrrggggghhhhhh!*" He's thrashing around. Kidd calls in more men from security.

"Mike, hey Mike! We're putting a tube down your throat."

"No, get that thing out of my mouth. Get it out of my nose! Get it out of my nose!"

Six men are now holding Mike down. He's sliding all over the exam table, slipping in his own blood from the accident. A bright red stream pours out of his nose. Kelly has come in to help Kidd jam in the tube. Mike is screaming about somebody named Ruth as the six attendants and nurses try to wrestle him down. "Ruth! Protect me. It's going down my nose hole. Somebody protect me. My nose. You're trying to kill me. Stop right now."

Kidd, who seems to be teaching Kelly some of the finer points about inserting an NG tube on a writhing patient, orders the attendants to strap on leather four-point restraints.

"I can't breathe. I can't breathe."

"Swallow now," shouts Kelly.

"Swallow," says Kidd, frustrated. "You're a real animal, Mike, you know that?"

For several minutes, the two residents struggle with Mike, ignoring the other accident victims, including the driver of the pickup, who had been unconscious. As an observer, I say nothing, though I felt the apprehension of the formidable-looking nurse. When were the doctors going to help the other people? What were they doing? Why was it so damn important to get in that tube?

In fact, said Tom Kirsch, an emergency medicine and trauma specialist at Johns Hopkins, inserting an NG tube at this stage of the workup was "useless" and certainly not important enough to be spending several minutes trying to get in while ignoring other seriously injured patients. "If this guy was in that severe of an MVA [Motor Vehicle Accident]," said Kirsch, "and was intoxicated and combative, there are a lot of things you do before you put the NG tube in. It's of minimal benefit in traumas. It's way down the list in the ATLS

[Advanced Trauma Life Support] protocol." When I read this comment to Kidd, he disagreed. Inserting an NG tube was the protocol in his hospital for all trauma victims, he said. "It's like drawing blood; it's part of the workup." But he admitted that he and Kelly had been overly concerned with this procedure that day. "We were new at this," he said. "We didn't have the judgment to know."

Later, Kelly explained that a few days earlier, he and Kidd were on duty when physicians in the main E.R. had failed to place an NG tube into a drunk, convinced he was not seriously hurt. Later that night a CAT scan showed his spleen had ruptured, which bounced him over to trauma, and a trip to the O.R. for emergency surgery. "Did we maybe over-learn that lesson?" said Kidd, who finally ordered a "huge hit" of Ativan and Haldol to sedate Mike. "Maybe. Maybe. It's hard to know."

■

No objective data exists on how often residents get in over their heads. But at the very least, my stint with the "bad boys" suggests what might go wrong in a system that purposely drops young physicians into complex, intense situations with minimal training. It also exposes the weakness of a teaching philosophy so biased toward experience that educators and senior physicians are willing to take a chance that a night like this, or worse, might happen.

This is not how proponents of the traditional system characterize it. "The goal of our program is to train a person once and for all almost automatically how to move effectively into managing a medical problem, a medical emergency," says John Potts, Chief of Internal Medicine at Boston's Massachusetts General Hospital. His program is well known for placing interns in the midst of a busy ward from the moment they begin their training, giving them maximum responsibility with minimal interference by attendings—something Potts and others call "invisible supervision." This hands-off style of education is necessary, he says, to teach young doctors how to handle everything on their own. "The facts may change, the medicines may change, but that marvelous training of how to cope is what the training period's about, and I don't see how you can fundamentally change that."

This seems a reasonable theory, yet the reality is a system that has become so weighted toward education by doing—what Thomas Dewey called "experiential learning"—that the residency places little emphasis on formal and didactic teaching, or the notion that trainees need to be closely, even intimately, watched and preceptored by senior doctors. For years, residents and educators have used a term for this method of teaching—"See one, do one, teach one," a concept I shall call the "plunge-in method."

I can think of no better illustration than what happened that balmy night in Trauma 3, when a brand new PGY3, with twenty-four months of experience, was left to teach and directly supervise a novice who just a month earlier had been handed his M.D., and was still getting used to being called "Doctor." Indeed, not only were these two tenderfoots responsible that night for Mike and the six other crash victims, over the course of their twenty-four-hour shift they treated thirteen other medium to severe trauma patients and numerous cuts and bumps, the biggest rush coming between 2:15 A.M. and 4 A.M. They were also responsible for managing eight post-trauma patients on the surgical wards, some in intensive care. These included a man in his early twenties shot three times in the belly; a drug dealer beaten up by a rival dealer with a 2 by 4; a "brain bleeder" hit by a car; two attempted suicides—one drank a six pack of beer, swallowed several Valium, and crashed into a wall while driving his car; the other leaped off an overpass—and another car accident victim with a crushed spleen. Finally, they were expected to help in the E.R. and in the O.R., if a patient was banged up enough to require surgery and they weren't needed elsewhere.

During their twenty-four-hour shift, the action ebbed and flowed. Once, between 9 P.M. and 11 P.M., it was so slow that Kidd threatened to break a long department tradition in the surgeons' lounge by drinking out of a blue mug—one of four colors of plastic cups for coffee. "No, not that!" said Claude, only half joking. He hadn't been here long, but he knew that no surgeon so much as touched a blue mug, which legend claimed would bring bad luck. Sure enough, when Kidd poured a steaming cup of ugly black coffee at 11 P.M. into a dusty blue mug, the team's beepers went off almost immediately. Later, in the thick of the mayhem, Kelly angrily chided Kidd: "You and your goddamned blue mug." Later, Kidd told me he will never touch a blue mug again.

Briefly, at about 1 A.M., the activity slowed enough for Kidd and

Kelly to sleep for a few minutes, before being summoned again to the trauma bays.

By 7 A.M., when their shift was almost over, the "bad boys" looked exhausted. "That was a bad night," said Kidd, rubbing his eyes. "We had it all at once. The worst thing is I was so tired, I lost track of who the patients were. They were all there, lined up, and I kept getting them mixed up."

■

It was the plunge-in method that allowed the PGY1 who splattered blood on me to attempt a central-line without supervision, having done it only a few times before. It is also why a surgical intern I met was permitted to fumble four different attempts at inserting a breathing tube before a senior resident showed her how to do it right. And it was the plunge-in method that contributed to Mary Allen's unfortunate demise.

"To call this education is wrong," says Bertrand Bell of the Bronx's Albert Einstein. "When people finish medical school, they can't take care of a cat. But they're expected to know everything in medicine on the first day they start as an intern. They are left as the front line to tend the patients, and they know next to nothing that's not in a book. This is madness."

Of course, interns don't issue forth completely unprepared. In medical school, they spend at least a year rotating through major departments in affiliated hospitals, observing and participating in patient care. How seriously this training is taken by each hospital varies enormously, however. In the best programs, during third year "clerkships" students are given responsibility to manage one or two patients for a few days alongside the residency team—an excellent method to launch the transition from classroom to clinic. Yet in one of the worst examples of the plunge-in method, many programs delegate an already overwhelmed intern to serve as primary tutor to the medical student. This all but guarantees a less than satisfactory third-year experience, and too often becomes an introductory course in See One, Do One, Teach One. On many nights, I watched beleaguered interns *start* their instruction of a medical student working on a patient long after midnight, when both teacher and student were exhausted—and patients had to be awakened to again give histories and be examined. Other times, interns simply ignored their medical student, having no time for them, period.

Every July, the obvious defects of this system manifest when interns arrive in hospitals, fresh from medical school—and residency directors and attendings complain about the lack of practical skills among their new recruits. "We have expanded our orientation to a whole week," said one director, "because we get starting interns in here who don't even know how to use a stethoscope, or take a history." What is astonishing about this remark is that this director, like many I talked to, seems oblivious to one of the chief reasons why: that fledgling clinicians cannot possibly learn efficiently from fledgling clinicians.

■

In past centuries, the most conscientious physician trainees learned the skills of their profession by apprenticing to an older physician, and not by plunging in. Initially they swept floors and performed nursing duties, as a mentor/instructor gradually taught them how to grind and mix drugs, diagnose disease, take histories, and, as medical knowledge advanced, to thump the abdomen and feel a pulse. Even though medicine was primitive and the knowledge base minuscule compared to today, it typically took many years of close instruction (and fees paid to a teacher) before an apprentice physician was recognized as a master who could practice competently on his own—and was allowed by reputable physicians and hospitals to work independently on patients.*

Not every physician was trained this way, particularly in mid-nineteenth-century America, where rules requiring hands-on training for physicians were sometimes lax, and where many physicians received degrees from schools that made little effort to teach practical medicine, offering a thick didactic soup of books and classroom lectures. Indeed, the idea of an immersion into a hands-on style of training—championed by William Osler of Johns Hopkins, the Mayo brothers in Minnesota, and other physician-innovators in the late nineteenth century—was itself a reaction against an educa-

*By late nineteenth-century America, medical education typically consisted of two years of classroom instruction and three of apprenticeship. In the absence of strict national standards, programs varied widely in the content and quality of their training.

tional system that was in many cases the opposite extreme to the plunge-in method.

Still, society has long demanded that inexperienced physicians stay clear of patients, or approach them only under close supervision. Almost since writing was invented, countless edicts, corpi, laws, codes, treatises, and admonitions share a common theme—that unseasoned doctors are a "plague on humanity," in the words of Samuel Johnson, and should never be allowed to work on patients without proper training and supervision.

Two and a half millennia ago, in the corpus attributed to the famous Greek physician Hippocrates, he (or one of his followers) writes that "Inexperience . . . is a cursed treasure and store for those who have it, whether asleep or awake; it is a stranger to confidence and joy, and a nurse of cowardice and of rashness." Hippocrates adds: "Let one of your pupils be left in charge, to carry out instructions," but only "those who have already [been] admitted into the mysteries of the art, so as . . . to give treatment with safety."

In the mid–thirteenth century, Holy Roman Emperor Frederick II issued an edict condemning the "irreparable suffering which may occur as a consequence of the inexperience of physicians." He ordered all doctors to study humanities for three years at a university, attend medical school for another three years, and pass an exam. Before being licensed, "he shall not practice medicine until he has during a full year devoted himself to medical practice with the advice and under the direction of an experienced physician"—a year apparently being enough to master what little medicine was known in the Middle Ages. Frederick also ordered that medical schools in his domains "teach not only theoretic, but also practical medicine." The penalty for violating this edict was "confiscation of goods, and a year in prison."

As recently as the early nineteenth century, administrators at Massachusetts General Hospital in Boston felt compelled, when asking the state for funds, to reassure state legislators that they had no intention "to give to students in medicine an opportunity to experiment, at the expense of the feelings, health, and lives of the poor patients." Insisting that the "inconvenience" to patients and to the smooth running of the hospital was at risk if trainees were allowed to roam about unattended, the statement banned trainees from talking to nurses or patients—and to each other when on the wards or in the O.R. These admonitions applied specifically to medical students, since there were no residents in the modern sense; yet they suggest a common trepidation about allowing tenderfoot doctors to work on patients.

Indeed, this century's dramatic volte-face from the fears of the past was motivated in part by a new educational imperative to standardize a vigorous curriculum, and to provide doctors-to-be a more practical, hands-on experience. But it also involved a more pragmatic reality that developed as hospitals grew in the late nineteenth and early twentieth centuries from charity hospices manned mostly by private doctors and their apprentices to large hospital-research complexes offering the latest in high-tech medicine. Suddenly, there was a need for more physicians to cover the rapidly expanding wards—particularly as senior physicians in hospitals slowly withdrew from active management of floor patients to conduct research and to see ever more patients in their clinics and private offices.

Residents filled the gap. According to sociologist Paul Starr, writing in his Pulitzer Prize–winning book, *The Social Transformation of American Medicine,* attendings and hospitals by the 1940s realized they could double and triple their patient load (and revenues) if they left most of the work to residents, who were then paid little more than room and board. Attendings were also freed up to conduct research, and to bring in lucrative grants to fund projects (and new facilities) for everything from cancer to heart disease. In other words, economics and convenience played as much a role in establishing the plunge-in system as did education, despite those educators who insist it is the only way to learn medicine properly.

Soon enough, it became virtually a religion as the rigor, intensity, autonomy, and self-sacrifice inherent to the plunge-in method evolved into a revered ritual by fire for successive generations of trainees—mostly men whose sense of camaraderie and bonding was forged by an experience many compared to boot camp in the army.

That most survived the ordeal intact, and emerged as competent physicians, seemed to verify both the method and the madness— and further cemented the hold of the plunge-in method in the imagination of modern educators and physicians. Indeed, one is tempted to describe the sanctity and exclusivity of this system, and the claim that it is good for patients, as a medical version of Plato's Myth of the Metals, where the rulers of the Republic maintain order by telling everyone they are born of gold, silver, or copper, those of gold being destined to rule; those of silver being destined to serve as administrators, soldiers, and merchants; and those of copper being foreordained to be laborers, farmers, and servants. This "noble lie" is perpetuated for the greater good, insists Plato. But here the similarity with the modern medical residency ends. For Plato in *The Republic* assumes that his philosopher-rulers understand the myth is a myth. In medicine, this has not always been the case. Only recently has the possibility that the old imperative might be more myth than reality occurred to reformers—and, when pressed, to a few old-line educators.

This reminds me of a department chairman I first met three years ago. For over an hour, he discussed in detail everything that was wrong with the old-fashioned residency, and why fundamental change was necessary, only to implore me at the end not to mention any of this to his residents. "I would appreciate it if you don't tell them we want to dramatically change the program," he said, "because what happens then is house staff come up here and say 'Don't change it, don't change it.' This is because you work so hard, so that your ego cannot take the bruising that would result if you admitted that you are spending all this effort and going to all this sacrifice if the program wasn't top-notch, if it is not the best way to learn medicine."

Three years later, most of the changes he proposed remain unmade. The house staff in his department continue to operate under the modern residency's great myth—that their method of training is hallowed, their self-sacrifice always justified, and whatever suffering is inflicted on patients is either unavoidable, or inherent to learning medicine. This is what Jim Stern believed, and Claude Kelly, and Bill Kidd.

Traditional educators are correct when they insist that young physicians cannot learn medicine without *doing* medicine, just as pilots cannot learn to fly without actually flying, and journalists cannot write stories without actually putting pen to paper. They miss the point, though: that the plunge-in method, like so much else in medicine, has taken a reasonable proposition that Hippocrates and Frederick II would undoubtedly have agreed with, and pushed it so far that its usefulness is often lost in excess. As Drs. Kelly and Kidd unwittingly illustrate, it also is potentially dangerous for patients—particularly in an acute situation like major trauma in the middle of the night.

■

By eight o'clock on that hot morning in July, the trauma rooms were quiet, and Kidd and Kelly were about to sign out their patients to the other surgical trauma team on call that month. Sitting down with Greg Maines, one of the chief residents, they reviewed what happened the night before, drinking coffee and eating poppyseed cakes in a lounge near the E.R. Maines, a short, muscular fifth-year resident who was headed for a fellowship in neurosurgery the following year, listened as Kidd talked about Mike the van driver and the bedlam in the trauma rooms around three A.M. "What you're telling me is you guys were in over your heads," said Maines, biting into a cake. "You should have called someone."

"The chief was in the O.R. with a triple A," said Kidd nonchalantly, meaning that the fifth-year in-house supervisor had been busy with an abdominal aortic aneurysm—a sudden swelling at the base of the aorta, where it divides in the abdomen into two branches, one headed into each leg. Allowed to distend unchecked, a "triple A" can rupture and kill a patient within minutes.

"So why didn't you call the SICU resident?" asked Maines, his tone less congenial than before.

"Fuck 'em," said Kidd, dismissing the comment with another of his ironic grins. "What would they know?"

"Then you should have called me," said Maines, clearly unhappy with Kidd's attitude.

"Get out of here," said Kidd.

"Really. You shouldn't be doing all of that on your own."

■

Except for Maines's comments over cake and coffee, there were no reprimands, no soul-searching over the potential hazards to patient care, no discussion of whether or not the events in Trauma 3 represented a fundamental flaw in the training. Mike the van driver and the others survived, but as Maines later told me, "It could have been worse."

Recently, Kidd's program did add a layer of supervision with a requirement that the PGY3 in trauma inform the attending on call about all level-one cases coming into the E.R., though this procedure is usually done over the phone. The PGY5 "chief" is also supposed to check on level-one traumas, though both the call to the attending and the look-see by the chief typically occur after the initial emergency. This frequently means the junior residents are still in charge during the critical first phase of a trauma situation.

Taking to heart Maines's criticism, Kelly told me he would try to call in help sooner next time. "But it's sometimes hard to know in the middle of everything when to do this," he said. As for Kidd, he still thought the night had been a good learning experience. "It was great handling all of that on my own," he said.

Yet this young disciple of the plunge-in method seems to be missing the greatest lesson of all about what happened that night in Trauma Room 3—*that he didn't know what he didn't know.*

CHAPTER 3

A Working Knowledge

The sum total of medical knowledge is now so great and widespreading that it would be futile for any one man . . . to assume that he has even a working knowledge of any large part of the whole.

William J. Mayo, M.D., 1910

For years, the plunge-in method worked well enough—in large part because it was possible for one person to learn most of what was known about medicine. Expectations remained low among physicians and the public that medicine could cure and treat most disease. As late as the 1940s, the corpus of medical knowledge was still manageable—at least compared to today. "In those days, people just died," said seventy-three-year-old Robert Nye, a retired physician and physiologist at Dartmouth who trained in the 1940s. "Unlike today, this was accepted, since there was a general understanding that doctors had no real treatments for most illnesses."

Consider that most dramatic and well-known procedure known as "code blue." Called when a patient's heart stops, a "code" in many people's minds is the ultimate symbol of modern medicine's frenzied but unflappable reaction to an emergency in which seconds count, and the failure to restore a heartbeat will cause brain damage and then death within minutes. Yet as ubiquitous as the "code" has become (television's *E.R.* runs an average of three a show, by my informal count), it may surprise many people that this procedure was not perfected and widely used until the mid-1960s. For most of this century, and before, when someone's heart stopped, it either started up again on its own, or the person died.

This was the state of affairs one night in 1948, when Robert Nye was a twenty-six-year-old medicine intern at Strong Memorial Hospital in Rochester, New York, checking on a dying patient. Bunched around the bed in a bare, four-person ward costing a paying patient

$15 a day, the man's wife and grown children sullenly waited for the end. Nye describes himself as being lean with angular cheeks, dressed in a white doctor's frock with a vicar-style collar snapped shut on one side.

In those days, says Nye, no machines whirred or beeped, and no air conditioners hummed to cool a room sweltering in a summer heat wave. There was no call button, television, or electronic control for raising and lowering the bed. Glass I.V. bottles hung beside the patient, regulated by a one-cent metal clamp pinching rubber tubes. In a deep, British-accented voice—Nye spent most of his childhood in London—he asked the family how they were holding up as he took the patient's pulse. The heart beat weakly, but at a regular rate. "For some reason," Nye said, "I kept my finger on the pulse as we talked. As I held it there, it suddenly stopped. I calmly finished whatever I was saying, and asked the family if they would kindly go outside for a moment. I then went and got myself a syringe—they were glass in those days—and a small-bore needle about four inches long. I filled it with epinephrine* and stuck it through the chest into the man's heart." Nye says he waited to see if this stimulant would work. When it didn't, he found the family and delivered the bad news. "And that," says Nye, "was a 'code blue' in the nineteen-forties."

■

Flash ahead forty-five years to Rhode Island Hospital in Providence. It's midmorning in April 1993, and I'm walking down a corridor on the seventh floor of the main hospital with Peg Miller, a thirty-one-year-old medicine intern I've been following on call since early the previous day. Over the intercom comes an announcement: "Blue team, 7B. Blue team, 7B."

To most nonmedical people in the corridor, these words mean nothing. Years ago, most hospitals stopped announcing "code blue" or "code red" because it frightened patients and families. But Peg Miller knew. Though postcall—she had been on duty some twenty-six hours, and was not officially assigned to that day's "blue team" handling codes—she was already on the seventh floor. "We're close," she said, picking up her pace. "Let's go see if we can help."

*Epinephrine stimulates the autonomic nervous system (involuntary "fight or flight" responses); it is used to assist in resuscitating a victim of cardiac arrest.

Thirty seconds later, she arrived outside 7B's Intermediate Respiratory Care Unit (IRCU, pronounced "UR-QUE"), where post–intensive care patients come to be weaned from respirators. A few minutes earlier, a nurse noticed a sixty-seven-year-old end-stage cancer patient's heart had stopped. (Since leaving the medical intensive care unit he had not been monitored via the central telemetry screens at the nurse's station, because he seemed to be improving). Calling a code, she had begun CPR while other nurses wheeled in the "crash cart." This looks something like a master mechanic's tool chest, stuffed with everything a code team is likely to need to perform an Advanced Cardiac Life Support (ACLS) protocol—drugs, syringes, I.V. bags, monitors, electrode leads for the EKG, and a charged defibrillator for shocking the heart. Already, nurses had hung plastic I.V. bags, regulated by beeping regulators flashing dosages and flow times in glowing red numbers.

As in most teaching hospitals, this code is resident led, with assistance from nurses, who sometimes know the protocol better than the young doctors. The prospect of leading a code—which first happens at Rhode Island during a resident's second year—terrifies most residents. "The first code I led," said a PGY2 at Rhode Island, "I didn't have any idea what I was doing. I found myself asking this nurse what to do about every fifteen seconds. Without her, I would have blown it."

As Peg Miller enters the room, Carolyn McGrath, the resident directing the code, is reading the EKG and other monitors as nurses finish affixing electrodes to the man's chest. His nightshirt has been ripped away, revealing skin so white it's almost translucent, and fine white hairs like cilia standing on end from static electricity. His chest is still. The room is filling up fast—I count seventeen people, including nurses, residents, and techs. By the end, over twenty people will crowd a room slightly larger than a one-car garage.

"Looks like a v-fib," says McGrath, meaning a ventricular fibrillation. This is when there is no pulse, but the heart is twitching. "Give him a milligram of epi," shouts McGrath over the din of activity. She's referring to epinephrine, the same stimulant injected by Bob Nye forty-five years earlier. This time, the "epi" is not dispensed with a needle plunged into the heart, to avoid poking holes in delicate tissue. These days the epi is injected into the femoral artery near the groin, chosen because this vessel's big, easy to reach in an emergency, and linked directly to the heart.

McGrath shouts to Peg Miller to draw blood so they can test the patient's "blood gases"—measurements of oxygen, carbon dioxide, and pH. Peg snatches a needle from the cart and draws a vial of dark red liquid from the femoral. Almost before it's full, a nurse is snatching it away to run it to the lab, five floors down. She shouts into an intercom on the wall with an open channel to 7B's nursing station, asking the clerk to let the hospital's lab know a code blood gas is coming. Others shout to the clerk to get electrolytes "stat."— quickly—and to run a full Chem 7, a blood test that measures electrolytes, creatinine, BUN, and glucose. Another intern inserts a more permanent needle and plastic line into the femoral, so "epi" and other drugs can instantly flow into the bloodstream.

McGrath, with short blond hair and a round, young-looking face that belies her age—she's in her midthirties and has come to medicine late—yells for everyone to stand clear. She grabs the two disks of the defibrillator. "Prepare to shock!" she shouts, placing the disks on the patient's chest. When she punches the buttons in the handles, the man's entire body quakes with the force of 200 joules of electricity.

"Pulse!" shouts McGrath, calm and confident. Near the end of her three-year residency, she is running the code because the second-year resident carrying the blue team beeper is busy elsewhere. Undeniably, she is good, a case in point that the residency system, at least as it's practiced at Rhode Island, produces competent physicians by the time they finish their three years. Later, after the code, McGrath's cool would dissolve as she sat wearily in a window well and dejectedly told me this man should never have received a code. "He is terminal," she said. "He should be DNR. But the family did not give consent, so we had to run the code. What a waste of time. But we have to go full bore, even if we don't think it's right."

"Nothing yet," yells a nurse. Someone else is shouting something about lidocaine; another voice says, "*ten* milligrams. It should be *ten* milligrams." Yet another is telling McGrath about the patient's cardiac history. "Oh yeah, and he has renal failure."

"We'll talk about that later." McGrath cuts her off. "Now, prepare to shock!"

McGrath pushes the buttons. The body jerks higher, hanging in midair for an instant as it quivers, juiced up this time with 300 joules.

"We have a pulse!" someone shouts.

"Pressure?" asks McGrath.

"Stand by. It's there. It's there, 180 over 120."

"Yes," someone cries, with the unrestrained relief of a soldier who has taken a hill and made it alive. "We got it! We got it!"

∎

How can anyone possibly measure the distance covered between these two "codes"? Between a lone intern injecting a single drug into a man quietly slipping away, and twenty specialists screaming and straining in a crisis mode similar to a battlefield as they bring to bear a dizzying array of machines, drugs, and know-how. And what about the ethical murkiness of saving a cancer patient at the end of his life? This was something that never even crossed the mind of Bob Nye half a century ago.

Listing what is new since 1948 would take thousands of pages, maybe tens of thousands.* *Open heart surgery. Magnetic Resonance Imager. Intensive care units. Percutaneous transluminal coronary angioplasties. DNA mapping. Ventilators. Legal abortion. Surfactant. Electrocauterization. Cephalosporins. Artificial hips, knees, elbows, hands, arms, and legs. Test tube babies. Pagers. Vaccines for polio, measles, rabies, and flu.*

How many millions of years have been collectively added to American lives? How many new treatments and diseases—and complications—are being discovered and perfected at this very moment?

Patients admitted to hospitals today are far sicker than in 1948, as lesser ailments once treated in-house are dealt with in outpatient clinics—everything from angioplasties (opening up clogged heart vessels by inserting and inflating a special balloon) to kidney dialysis. "Patients are sicker and more complicated than they used to be," says Mark Fagan, the director of Rhode Island's Medical Primary Care Unit, and Peg Miller's attending. He is talking about when he was a resident in the early eighties, just a dozen years ago. "The number of interventions per patient is higher now," he says,

---

*In 1973, Herrman Blumgardt, a renowned physician and researcher at Harvard, suggested that medical science discovered or invented an average of 500 drugs a year. If that's true, since 1973 some 10,000 new drugs alone have been added to medicine's fund of available pharmaceuticals.

"so is the level of precision treatment you have to think about. For example, when I trained it was very rare to have a patient on a vent[ilator] outside of the unit. I mean it was one a year. We residents would kick and scream and jump up and down if they had a patient on a vent on their floor." Now vents are everywhere on the wards, he says.

"Recently, I looked at *Harrison's Principles of Internal Medicine*," adds Lucian Leape, who trained as a surgeon in the early sixties. "It's twice as fat as it was when I studied. You look at *Principles of Bio-Chemistry*—it's twice as big as it was when I studied. The amount of information that doctors are supposedly supposed to know is at least twice, and probably ten times as much as it was when I graduated from medical school, and we thought it was pretty hard to assimilate at that time." Other educators suggest a doubling every five to ten years.

Meanwhile, hospitals have grown into small cities, with some academic centers covering several blocks. They employ thousands, and spend hundreds of millions of dollars a year, even as the government and insurance companies clutter physicians' desks, answering machines, and hard drives with ever more bureaucratic demands and oversight requirements.

In 1940 there were 5,000 residents on the rolls at fewer than 600 hospitals in the United States. Today almost 100,000 residents and fellows train at 1,223 teaching hospitals. Even more recent is a seismic shift from the days when medical schools graduated almost exclusively young, single white males, with only a scattering of women, older students, and minorities. In the 1970s this abruptly shifted, in part because white males suddenly switched from medicine to other professions. At the same time, medical schools and residency programs were wildly expanding. This meant a sudden rise in the number of nontraditional physicians, with the population of doctor-trainees shifting from more than 90 percent white and male in the 1960s to 30 percent women and 18 percent minorities today.

Nearly half of all house officers are married; many of these have children during a training stint that has grown from an average of one year in the 1940s to a minimum of five years for surgeons, four years for OB–GYNs, and three years for internal medicine and pediatrics. For some specialties, physicians rack up as many as a dozen years mastering, say, plastic surgery and certain cardiothoracic techniques.

The sum of these tectonic dislocations is an immeasurable upsurge in intensity for those at the fulcrum of medicine—physicians—who still are expected to be on top of every new development, computer protocol, Diagnostic Rating Group, contraindication, and procedure. For older physicians, the transformation has been particularly dramatic compared to when they trained, though they at least have absorbed change over time—unlike residents, who are expected to learn everything all at once.

"It was an easier time to be a resident," says Bob Nye about the forties. "We worked the same hours as they do today, possibly more, but we just didn't have as much to do, or to know." Another physician who trained in the nineteen-forties, former AMA president Dr. John Tupper, an internist from the University of California at Davis, told me that a "call night" when he was an intern meant "you tucked in your patients at night and hoped they would be alive the next morning. Then you went to sleep." Tupper said that typically he would be awakened only if a new admission came in, or to pronounce a patient dead.

Despite this, one still hears frequently from older physicians that they worked harder when *they* trained—something Massachusetts General's John Potts, for one, says emphatically is not true. "There is an ill-advised tendency," he told me, "to say, 'Well, I did it, so you can do it.' My reaction to that is: rubbish. These young people are seeing much sicker patients, and they can offer many more modalities of treatment and therefore the stress of making a mistake is much higher than when I was a house officer twenty or thirty years ago."

■

Traditionalists among educators insist they are well aware of medicine's breathtaking pace of change, but they still staunchly believe in the old system—i.e., the plunge-in method. Indeed, they claim to have compensated for the crush of new information, and the stress of trying to learn and apply it all, by reducing call nights and, in some cases, patient loads. Others insist this is not enough—that modest alterations in call night schedules can not counteract the onslaught of technology. "Shaving off a couple of hours here and there hardly makes up for what is an entirely new world of medical care," said a former resident in California. Likewise, Harvard internist Timothy McCall has written that given the increase in what a resident needs to know, "Working hours will have to be decreased, if only to keep stress at present levels."

The only way to truly settle this would be to somehow measure the intensity per hour for individual residents—the number of decisions, orders, interactions, and inputs of data produced, say, every sixty minutes—and compare it to years past. But until this is done, if it can be, we'll have to depend on common sense to guide us as we consider whether Bob-Nye's residency in the forties, or Mark Fagan's in the early eighties, was more or less intense per hour than someone on call in Peg Miller's generation.

I asked Bob Nye about this. He says he carried a maximum of thirty-two patients at a time on the public wards, where his heart attack patient "coded." He also had to do most of his own lab work, draw blood, and sometimes do custodial work. Some forty-five years later, the interns I followed, including Peg Miller, carried an average of ten to twelve patients at a time, though some managed as many as fifteen and even twenty, with one internal medicine team at Duke—an intern, a resident, and a medical student—carrying twenty-one patients when I visited. (They complained mightily because the other team on their service had only seventeen patients). As for scut work, hospitals vary, but most still require residents to draw blood and to perform menial chores for at least part of the day.

Most of Nye's patients were not seriously ill, however. Nor could he do much technically to help. In contrast, interns today must cope with patients who demand up to several hours of individual attention each day, sometimes at the same time, when two or more "crash" and the intensity scale blasts through the roof.

"It's obviously detrimental to the learning process to have too many patients at once," admitted Mike Zabel, chief medical resident at Duke University Hospital in 1993. Sitting in a spare office down the hall from the hospital's medicine wards, he explained to me why his medicine program was shifting from every third night on call to every fourth—a move Zabel said the department heads were making reluctantly, convinced that the more hours spent in the hospital the better. Indeed, Zabel told me the new plan was motivated less by concern about stress and intensity than by the fact that Duke's patient admissions were rising—and the number of residents was not.

In 1988, when Zabel interned at Duke, he said PGY1's admitted an average of 5 patients per call night. (This was in addition to patients already under their care admitted on previous nights.) Now the number, he said, is an average of 6.4 admissions per call, with the patients much sicker. Switching to every fourth night will help drop the number back to five, he contended, and will reduce the overall patient load per resident.

Without a doubt, this will make things easier for Duke residents. But all it will really do (if it works) is return the gross number of patients back to the 1988 level, without compensating for the increases in knowledge, technology, and intensity of illness since Zabel's residency. "We will continue to chase the optimum number in the face of advancing technology," said Zabel. "We think we're getting it right. But who knows?"

■

Working conditions aside, there is also the matter of what does *not* get learned when such a high premium is placed on knowing what one educator called "ten pounds of facts squeezed into a five-pound bag." According to Bertrand Bell, an overemphasis on high-tech medicine and learning about every drug and treatment "leaves no space in a trainee-doctor's brain for the most important part of medicine, learning the c.s. factor—the common sense factor." Residents have trouble, insists Bell, knowing what to do, and devising plans of action, when a patient's symptoms deviate from a textbook diagnosis. "Say a patient has a dangerously high fever. As any mother knows, the first thing you do is cool them down," he says. "Only then you run the fancy tests and come up with what's wrong. What happens these days is they have to come up with a diagnosis before they act."

As the editor in chief of *The New England Journal of Medicine* put it in a recent editorial: "Technology is no substitute for careful clinical reasoning." Writing about the need to teach problem solving in an age of machines and an over-reliance on tests, Jerome P. Kassirer, M.D., said that it is critical for physicians to master the age-old art of diagnosis by learning how to think, not by "mindlessly ordering one test after another in the hope that the correct diagnosis will emerge."

Robert Nye agrees, saying with his trademark deep chuckle that perhaps his generation got at least one thing right. "Because we didn't have all this technology cluttering things up," he said, "we were able to focus far more on the art of medicine—on how to interact with patients, and how to solve basic problems. We depended a lot more on common sense. Wouldn't it be nice if we could bring back that part of the old-fashioned training of my day, and realize it is probably as important to being a good doctor as all the great technologies of the past fifty years?"

CHAPTER 4

Signing Off

They give up too much responsibility. They leave us alone
too much. But I enjoy it.

Surgical resident

Three times that day—a Thursday—Dr. Rich Ferrara, a PGY4 in anesthesiology,* pitched in to help an exhausted PGY2 in the O.R. Almost from the beginning, the operation had gone badly. As surgeons cut and dissected, trying to repair a forty-seven-year-old woman's damaged L-3 vertebra—the third vertebra down in the lower (lumbar) section of the back—the resident struggled to keep the patient stable. But surgeons kept nicking blood vessels running alongside the spine, causing massive blood losses the anesthesiologists frantically replenished—at a rate of almost six units of whole blood an hour.†

"This was a forty-seven-year-old lady who was struck by a car several weeks earlier, who fractured her third lumbar vertebra," explains Ferrara, a short man with deep olive skin, wavy black hair, and a cool and composed style of speaking. "It was still damaged, because these injuries don't always heal well, so she was coming in electively to have it repaired. She was an active person, a runner and hiker, and since the accident she had not been able to do these things." Called a lumbar corpectomy, this procedure takes a damaged vertebra and replaces the weakened, shattered bone with something hard and rigid, like metal, so the patient can regain some use of their back.

"It started out routine, then it just sort of went bad," Ferrara recalls, drinking a cup of coffee several months later. As he speaks a look of great sadness comes over him, a reticence greatly at odds with

---

*Anesthesiology residents spend their PGY1 year as interns in either a general surgery or general medicine program. They are then required to complete three years of anesthesiology training.
†A unit of blood equals 250 cc; five units equals the entire amount of blood in a typical adult human. This amount is called a "blood volume."

74

his usual aplomb. His words spill out in a monotone. "These cases can be bloody, but this one was especially bloody. They had the woman up on her side. They went in through her back and they dissected down to the level of the spine, and they were pushing away the nerve roots and the arteries and veins that feed the cord itself. Corpectomies are never pretty, but this one was extraordinarily bad."

At seven P.M., with the surgeons still operating after eleven hours, Ferrara plunged in a fourth time. "I walked into the room," he says, "and saw that the surgery seemed to be wrapping up." As he took over monitoring vital signs and drug flows, and grabbed sacks of dark red blood to "push" into the patient, Ferrara noticed that the attending surgeon had gone, leaving a first-year orthopedic fellow to close up. This is common, he says, though attendings are required to stay in the hospital until a case is actually finished.

As the fellow and a surgical resident sewed suture into the first of several damaged blood vessels, the patient's blood pressure suddenly crashed. "It dipped down to about 55 over 30," says Ferrara, despite an epinephrine drip he had started to support the woman's pressure. (A normal b.p. should be about 120 over 80.) "I told the surgeons at that point that they had about thirty seconds to finish, because we were going to lose the patient if we didn't do something to restore her pressure."

The surgeons agreed and hastily closed; they then helped Ferrara adjust the operating table, moving the patient's head down to get blood into her brain. By now—it was about eight P.M.—the woman was teetering on a cardiac arrest as the team desperately tried to pump in blood to boost her pressure. Restoring a feeble but stable pulse, the surgeon announced he wanted to put a chest tube in before they finished. "This is commonly done when they're afraid they may have nicked the diaphragm," says Ferrara, "or gone through the diaphragm and nicked the pleura around the lung, which can cause some of the lung to collapse. This tube is placed preventively into the pleura on the outside of the lung in order to suck out any of the air that shouldn't be in there. So the surgical fellow put a chest tube in. But he didn't get it right, and he put it right through the pleura and into the pulmonary artery. This is the artery that comes out of the right ventricle, so the right heart was now pumping into this chest tube, and we suddenly had blood coming out everywhere, just when we were trying to resuscitate. He meant to just stick it in the pleura, but he wasn't supervised when he was doing this and he put it into the pulmonary artery, and so it was just very frightening and it was very obvious that we could not resuscitate.

"Somebody grabbed a bucket to catch all the blood, but then it was going all over the floor. They clamped it off very quickly, and we began CPR, and brought in the defibrillator because she went into very dangerous heart rhythms." When the team threaded a wire-guided catheter down the patient's esophagus they discovered that "her right heart had stopped pumping any blood, and was filling up and getting enormous and the left heart was empty. And she died. Despite our efforts, she died.

"But this was not the end of it," said Ferrara, staring off into space. "We had to go talk to the patient's family and explain to them what had been going on all these hours. We wanted the attending surgeon to be the one to do this, but he wasn't in the hospital. We paged him and paged him, and he didn't answer, and we called his home and his baby-sitter told us that he was out for the evening with his wife and couldn't be reached.

"He apparently thought it was a routine closure, even though this had been such a long case and the patient had needed so much in the way of blood replacement during the day. She was definitely on the edge, but until that last point she was maintaining stable vital signs." The attending, he says, should never have left with her still bleeding like that. "Then he was unavailable—which was unbelievable."

Ferrara says he had to notify the family, which should never have happened. "They were furious," he said. "They wanted to see the attending surgeon. They wanted to know who we were because they had never met us before. We were not the anesthesiologists they had met during pre-op. They were devastated, and the sad thing was the family was later convinced by the surgical fellow that came by and talked to them not to do an autopsy. They were told this was a natural, unforeseeable death in the O.R."

I asked if he agreed with this.

"Absolutely not," he said, his sadness shading into anger. "Basically, this was the way to save the surgeons' butts, because the autopsy would have shown there was a tube in the pulmonary artery and that would have looked terrible, so they allowed the patient to be taken to the morgue, and this mistake was buried with her, I guess."

∎

Rich Ferrara made it clear that this incident was isolated, that attending surgeons at his hospital seldom commit such errors of judgment, or engage in such apparent cover-ups. "This was the first and only time I saw this sort of cover-up happen," he said—prompting me to ask if I should even relate the story in this book. "You have to," he said matter-of-factly, "it's too important to ignore," a response that convinced me this anecdote was not solely about poor supervision, but about how a tragedy could permanently scar a talented young physician.

Nor is Rich Ferrara the only resident deeply affected by a horrific incident that might not have happened with proper supervision. "I had a friend doing a medicine residency who totally lost it one night," said a surgical intern on the West Coast. "At two A.M. he was alone, and he was off his floor getting a blood bag when a patient crashed. He came rushing back, and didn't know what to do, because the patient's pressure was falling, and he couldn't get in an I.V. He felt alone, flapping in the breeze. He was afraid to call his supervisor. The patient nearly died. He had a farc.* This was a caring guy. It really messed him up."

This same intern describes a night just a few days after he started his residency, when a patient on his service had a heart attack at two A.M. "There was no attending around," he said. "I was inserting one of my first central lines, and I popped [punctured] a lung. The R2 with me didn't have a clue. Here I was, this new intern, totally out of control. This patient might have died. Fortunately, she didn't. She stayed a few days longer and got a [chest] tube† she shouldn't have. This was a devastating experience for me." I asked if this incident was isolated, and the intern said: "We are constantly winging it."

I could go on. Indeed, many of the errors I've described so far would probably not have happened, or would not have been as serious, if supervision had been tighter.

"Most of the time," says Ferrara, "supervision is adequate. Sometimes it's excellent. But I've got to tell the truth. Bad things do happen because attendings are not around. Or they let a resident undertake a task beyond their experience. We see misadventures

---

* A heart attack.
† A chest tube to reinflate the lung.

quite a bit, especially in the middle of the night and in trauma situations." Usually, he says, someone more senior is around to save the situation—but not always. "I think they are allowed to do too much. They're given license to close patients and make decisions when they don't completely know what they're doing.

"Surgery is a very, very difficult thing to master," adds Ferrara. "We have some excellent surgeons who really care about teaching. Others don't. Those are the ones I try to avoid. Especially the cowboys who are too quick to cut." He says he has avoided the fellow who worked on the forty-seven-year-old woman. "I don't trust him," says Ferrara. "He's a cowboy."

■

Singling out the O.R. as an arena of poor supervision is not entirely fair. Physicians will tell you—and I have observed myself—that residents in O.R.s are probably the most closely supervised in the hospital, precisely because procedures like the one Rich Ferrara described are so complex and the downside so dramatic if errors are made.

If supervision breaks down among surgeons, it usually happens outside of the operating theater, on the wards. Surgical residents spend most of their first year taking care of postoperative patients on these floors, while attendings and more senior residents are busy in the O.R.'s. This is not to say that attendings don't care about their patients' postop. "The best surgeons almost care too much," says Bertrand Bell. "They are, after all, cutting into somebody. This makes them feel incredibly responsible for what happens to a patient after they close up the wound."

Despite this, attendings are seldom seen on the wards. Typically, they come in for lightening-quick rounds before heading to the O.R. in the morning, and again late in the day. Otherwise the surgical wards are the domain of interns, sometimes supervised by more senior residents (like Bill Kidd), and backed up by nurses who as often as not help fledgling PGY1's muddle through their first few crises.

"It's impossible to be in the O.R. and on the floor at the same time," notes Geena Carlson, a PGY2 in surgery. "Sometimes interns, who are inexperienced people, are left on the floor without any backup. In the middle of the day, just a busy day, the attendings are cranking out the patients [in the O.R.] and you're in charge of the step-down unit. You can have some pretty ill patients. No question. People are very much on the threshold, in the gray zone, and you really have to stay up on the details, and if an intern or resident isn't alert to those changes, you've got a mortality on your hands before you know it." She said this had never happened to her, but it did happen to another intern in her program, who mistakenly inserted a breathing tube into a forty-year-old asthmatic's esophagus instead of her windpipe. Carlson said that because everyone was busy elsewhere—in the O.R. and trauma rooms—the error was not caught for several minutes. The patient lives now "in a persistent vegetative state," according to another resident in the hospital.

"What you have [on the floor] is perhaps an intern surrounded by a bunch of nurses who albeit are very knowledgeable in terms of their experience," says Carlson. But they are not doctors, she explains, and don't always have the knowledge to grasp "the whole picture." Sometimes, she admits, the resident doesn't understand it either, a potentially disastrous combination that Carlson says could be alleviated by the presence of a senior resident or attending on the wards—not necessarily to treat patients, but as a resource. "Everybody should not be in the O.R. No way."

Surgery is hardly alone in sometimes overemphasizing the notion of "invisible supervision" on the wards. Internal medicine, pediatrics, OB–GYN, and other specialties also place a premium on having resident teams oversee floors while attendings (hopefully) monitor the action from afar, reading and signing off on charts, checking in on rounds, and returning pages when there are questions.

One specialty *has* emphatically decided to scrap the old system: emergency medicine. In recent years, E.R. physicians have aggressively transformed their arena from resident-controlled to one where an attending is *always* present, and *always* hands-on. This is a radical transformation from even the late 1980s, when E.R.'s were notorious as the least supervised service in most hospitals, directed on evenings and weekends (and sometimes during the day) almost exclusively by interns and junior residents. This meant that across America, E.R.'s at teaching hospitals were often manned by greenhorns less than two years out from medical school. (Millions of Americans watch the old system at work on the television series *E.R.*, which has residents running amok in a manner more like the early 1980s than the 1990s.) Emergency medicine's radical upgrade resulted in part from several highly publicized cases where patients were mishandled and hospitals sued. But even before this maelstrom of litigation, reformers for at least two decades had been philosophically urging a system by which residents would still operate independently but tethered to a very short leash—and with specially trained attendings ready to jump in at a moment's notice to salvage a deteriorating situation. Emergency physician Tom Kirsch of Johns Hopkins says there are still too many teaching hospitals without full-time coverage and supervision by emergency medicine specialists. "But it's a lot better than it was.

"Emergency medicine can be very intense," he adds, "with decisions that need to be made immediately by an experienced person. That's why we feel it's very important to have an attending there, to run things at all times." Kirsch says emergency medicine focuses first on the patient, and then on education—which he insists has *improved* the quality of instruction. "By any measure, we are turning out better emergency physicians than ever before," says Kirsch. "And we're maximizing safety for the patient." Of course, this system depends on senior physicians attending at night and on weekends—hours that attendings in other specialties seem unwilling to work routinely, too often leaving the wards during these off times to the residents and nurses.

■

As with most residency questions, data on supervision is spotty. According to a confidential study given to me by a resident in an East Coast hospital, 80 percent of the house staff in his department said they had experienced at least one or two episodes where patient care was "affected" by lack of supervision in a single month. Twenty percent said they had three to five incidents. Out of these, just under half the supervision incidents resulted in inconvenience or discomfort for the patient, one in ten triggered a minor complication, and one in thirty a major complication.

In 1993, researchers at the University of Florida at Jacksonville studied more than 4,000 surgical cases over the course of a year and found that the more an attending was present in the O.R., the lower the mortality and complication rates. In trauma cases, for instance, attendings scrubbed in and were present in 72 percent of the cases—and experienced a 26 percent mortality rate. In those cases where an attending did not scrub in, the mortality rate was almost a third higher. Complications that did not result in death were about 30 percent higher when an attending was not present.

In the thousands of pages of testimony, reports, and findings collected by the Bell Commission in 1987, other issues pale beside the paramount concern over supervision. According to Bell himself, supervision was always at the core of his committee's investigation—and the crux of the tragic death of a young woman in New York City that sparked the Bell hearings.

Her name was Libby Zion, an eighteen-year-old college freshman who arrived at New York Hospital's E.R. close to midnight on March 4, 1984. She presented with a high fever and an alarmingly high white blood cell count. She was also thrashing wildly for no apparent reason. Seven hours later, this previously healthy woman's temperature soared to 108 degrees. Her heart arrested, and she died. What exactly caused the fever remains a mystery, though in 1986 a grand jury noted in a blistering rebuke to the residency system that Libby Zion was never seen by a physician more senior than a second-year resident—a situation that was then considered normal and acceptable, and in many states still is.

"A hospital," wrote the grand jury, after holding twenty-four sessions and hearing twenty-two witnesses over a six-month period, "is not the place for recently graduated doctors to grow and develop in isolation; rather it is a place where the learning process should continue under strict supervision. Thus, medical decisions, whether in an emergency room or on a hospital floor, should not be made by inexperienced interns and junior residents without in-person consultations with more senior physicians."

Branding the residency system in New York as "counterproductive to providing quality medical care," and repleat with "serious deficiencies," the grand jury recommended that the state establish new regulations "to insure that interns and junior residents in level one hospitals are supervised contemporaneously and in-person by attending physicians or those members of the house staff who have completed at least a three-year postgraduate residency program. These regulations should narrowly define the circumstances under which interns may practice medicine without direct supervision."

   In the wake of this highly public finding, then state health commissioner Dr. David Axelrod created a blue ribbon committee composed of prominent physician-educators in New York—the Ad Hoc Advisory Committee on Emergency Services, the Bell Commission. Their recommendation echoed the grand jury, insisting that "there must be supervision in the hospital where there are residents in training in the acute care specialties . . . twenty-four hours a day, seven days a week, by licensed and currently registered physicians. . . . These physicians shall be present in person in the hospital to supervise the residents in their specific discipline and in sufficient numbers to meet reasonable and expected demand."

   In 1989, New York adopted these recommendations as law— along with other regulations governing graduate medical education. To date no other state requires twenty-four-hour supervision of all residents by statute.

■

   New York's laws were not enacted without a vigorous debate. For several days in August of 1987 representatives from state and national medical organizations converged in Albany and New York City to testify before Bell's committee in what remains the most public and comprehensive single airing ever on the medical residency— including what should be done, if anything, about the supervision question. Some of the witnesses testifying at the hearings supported the concept of increasing supervision. One of these was Paul Ebert, then director of the American College of Surgeons. He argued that a regulation for stepped-up supervision would not affect surgeons, since surgical attendings already watched their residents closely—at least in the O.R. Other physician groups conceded they could probably improve supervision in their programs, but they opposed any sort of mandatory rule. They also fretted about the cost of hiring additional attendings to increase supervision. Still others opposed the entire concept of the proposal, suggesting that residents in most situations were best "supervised" from a distance, using what a statement delivered by the American College of Physicians dubbed the principal of "Maximum control, minimum interference.

   "At the root of this principle," said this statement, "lies the recognition that the way residents gain competence and learn independent judgment [is] by working at the outer limits of their competence." Residents should be allowed to make as many decisions as possible by themselves, since "residents supervised too closely are at risk of emerging from training as useless or dangerous physicians . . . we've all seen such physicians: they over-use consultants, order excessive and inappropriate laboratory work, and have great difficulty responding to their patients' real emotional needs because they are so busy dealing with their own lack of confidence."

Few would disagree that physicians must learn to be coolheaded and decisive. "What you're learning is to be able to walk into a room and instantly understand what's going on," says Rich Ferrara, "and know exactly what's wrong or what's right and what needs to happen."

Yet to blame a physician's lack of confidence on too much supervision during his or her residency seems a stretch—particularly if that is the sole defense for a system where the "outer limits" of a resident's "competence" may mean putting a patient in harm's way. The College of Physicians' statement admits as much, noting "that residents will inevitably make some improper judgments." But they quickly dismiss this consideration with a sweeping generalization, and a strident insistence that it would be futile to tamper with the status quo. "There is no way around this problem," they declare, "short of eliminating residency training altogether."

Abolishing residencies is one way to solve the problem. Yet it seems one could reform the system short of this apocalyptic solution, so that residents—like junior pilots, nuclear power plant operators, and others who must learn a skill despite the danger of letting neophytes learn by experience—get the chance to make decisions on their own. The question is how to accomplish this without exposing patients to undue hazard.

■

Deciding when, and when not, to hold the hand of a young physician is hardly a new dilemma. Hippocrates emphasized that no pupil should "be left in charge, to carry out instructions . . . and to administer treatment" unless they "have been already admitted to the mysteries of the art," a process that he insisted should involve years of careful preparation under the intimate guidance of a teacher-physician. Galen, of ancient Rome, and leading Renaissance physicians also stress a careful, close period of direct, contemporaneous monitoring and instruction—an imperative that the unscrupulous and untalented frequently violated over the years, though it remained the ideal for hundreds of years, including the period early in this century when William Osler and others initiated the modern residency system. Indeed, even as the so-called medical giants revolutionized the way physicians were taught by full immersion into the wards, they assumed that novices would be guided by an intimate and constant interaction with elder teacher-physicians who knew practical medicine because they were seeing their own patients and keeping up with the latest treatments and research. "Osler made the hospital a medical school," writes medical historian Kenneth M. Ludmerer, "the students living and working in the hospital 'as part of its machinery, as an essential part of the work of the wards.' " Equally critical to this machinery, said Osler, was the teacher-supervisor. The student, he wrote, "learns under skilled direction when to act and when to refrain; he learns insensibly the principles of practice."

Osler and others of his generation may have championed the plunge-in method, but they never intended it to replace an active participation by clinical teachers—and the sort of mentoring and guidance that provides a careful balance between giving novices too much and too little responsibility. Here lies the essence of the problem today: that medical education has strayed dramatically from Osler's meticulous balance, shifting from the notion that teachers would also be scientists and clinicians to today's reality, where scientists and clinicians are also expected—sometimes grudgingly, and with little reward or encouragement from hospitals or peers—to squeeze in a little teaching.

In some ways, this reversal of Osler's arrangement was inevitable as hospitals expanded rapidly after Sir William's generation, and as attendings in the twenties and thirties slowly extricated themselves from the wards to pursue newfound passions. Eventually, as residents in midcentury subsumed the lion's share of the actual management of patient care, hospitals and faculty contrived the system in place today, in which attendings are almost always busy elsewhere, and residents scramble to decide when to stop the potassium drip for Mr. Smith, and if it's safe to turn off Mrs. Jones's ventilator, which could trigger cardiac arrest if done too early.

The core of this arrangement, called the chief resident system, is a theory that residents can and should be supervised day-to-day by more senior residents, with a chief resident in overall command. In medicine and pediatrics, the chief position is held for a year by someone who has just completed his or her residency. For surgery, the chief is usually a fifth-year resident. Attendings are not entirely absent, however, though their role is greatly diminished, with many on today's teaching hospital faculties devoting only a month or two on call each year. Even then, they typically spend only a few hours a week on the wards.

"After the Second World War," says Bertrand Bell, "the people who were on the faculty were not the people who were there to take care of the patients. They were there to do research and write papers—or to push papers as administrators." He contends that too many attendings today are really bench scientists who dislike their stints on the wards but are either forced to teach by contract or feel compelled by tradition. "They hate it," he says, "and they're even afraid of the responsibility, but we've got this ideal that an academic doctor is supposed to be a scientist and a clinician and a teacher"—something called "the triple threat." According to Bell, this has led to a "phenomenon . . . whereby residents feel they are responsible for patient care and in many ways consider the attending staff superfluous."

"I like medicine because it is a culture of learning," said a surgical intern, "but the instruction frequently comes from the least knowledgeable, the one just above you. You almost always have an attending checking your notes," he added. "And the good ones will spend time with you on attending rounds, asking good questions. But this completely depends on the [attitude of the] attending."

"I think that residents teaching residents is one of the great defects of the current system," agrees ethicist Edmund Pellegrino of Georgetown. "There is not enough supervision by the attending physician in the teaching process, or of the actions of the resident."

■

To find out exactly what the chief resident system was all about, I went to visit Steve Jones, the chief resident in Jim Stern's program. Like Stern, he was broad-chested and athletic looking, if slightly overweight—he said from "sitting around too much." Perched in his tiny cubicle of an office, which looked like a former closet, I asked him to give me a nuts-and-bolts overview of the system at his hospital. "Right now," he said, "we have probably three hundred medicine patients in the hospital, of which probably greater than 90 percent are covered by medical house staff." This is in a department with about 145 attendings and 75 residents, he explained—almost a two-to-one ratio. (Nationally, the ratio between faculty and medical students/residents hovers at about one to two.)

On the surface, this ratio suggests a phenomenal commitment to pedagogy—except that most of these 145 attendings' teaching duties, according to Jones, involve perhaps a lecture or two delivered each term at the medical school, along with one or two months of attending duties on the wards each year, and occasional meetings with advisees. The rest of their time has little or nothing to do with direct education.

"Some of these physicians whip in and out of town for conferences and meetings," mentioned Jones, talking about attendings. "They have grand rounds to give. They have heavy office responsibilities, and research, so it's difficult for them to watch their thirty patients who are very sick in the hospital and simultaneously be doing those other obligations." The house staff system allows them "to basically see two or three times more patients than they normally could, because if they had to go back and forth to go look at Mr. Smith every time Mr. Smith didn't feel well, they couldn't do what they normally do."

The few studies conducted on resident-attending interaction support the contention that attendings are not around much. One paper published in the *Journal of General Internal Medicine* found that interns while on call spent a mere 6.4 percent of their time with attendings—compared to 38.1 percent by themselves, 19.2 percent with resident supervisors, and 17.7 percent with patients. This is not to say that the chief resident system completely ignores residents on the wards or does nothing to prevent mistakes. In a good program, a hands-on residency director and chief resident will sometimes work almost as many hours as a resident designing curricula, organizing schedules, and troubleshooting when residents have problems—whether personal, ethical, or administrative.

"We try very hard here to get people who are all top-notch," says

Jones. "But clearly a small subset of people are not as good as the others. They either lack self-confidence, or other things"—a situation he says can drag down the rest of the team. If this happens, "we do various things. The chief resident or attending will sometimes tutor these people to help bring them up to speed. We change schedules to move people out of intense experiences into slightly less intense experiences." The chief might also ask nurses to keep an eye on a "weak link." But this happens only in extreme cases. Typically, explained Jones, the PGY2 in charge of each team has the "responsibility to make sure that the team runs smoothly, even if it means staying up very late to make sure intern x has all his bases covered." Still, after I detailed what happened with Mary Allen and other similar episodes, he admitted that some things can slip through the cracks. "It's not absolutely clear to me that it's the best way to do it."

I asked him if more attending time on the wards would help. Jones said it would. "But that would mean they would not have time to do their other things." Jones also suggested this would increase the cost of teaching residents—a point raised at the Bell Commission hearings by Jo Ivey Boufford, then president of the New York City Health and Hospitals Corporation, which administers New York's public hospitals. She estimated that for the eleven acute care hospitals, five chronic care hospitals, and more than forty ambulatory facilities governed at that time by the corporation, adding attending supervision twenty-four hours a day would cost between $19 million and $23 million extra per year. The actual cost of implementing New York's around-the-clock supervision rule—which went into effect in 1989—has never been determined, though annually the state and private insurers spend upwards of $200 million statewide to implement all of the Bell Regulations, including the provisions for increased supervision.

"I'm not sure anyone would design a system to work this way," said Steve Jones. "It's sort of the way it's evolved."

■

So the current system has embraced half of Osler's plan, but not the other half—upholding the idea of immersion and practical training, but failing to provide the deliberate mentoring and supervision the modern residency was founded upon. Even worse, this coincides with an era of profound shifts in technology and societal views of medicine, when young physicians more than ever need Osler's style of close instruction and guidance.

Possibly, this explains why some younger physicians are complaining they feel isolated from other doctors, particularly older, would-be mentors. "There's a sense that in the past, there was more of a connection between older and younger generations of doctors," said a young psychiatric attending in New York. "These days, there is none of this, which has left many of us feeling terribly alone."

Research verifies that most physicians today feel they have missed out on a meaningful mentoring experience, data that should alarm educators—if, in fact, the system as designed by Osler truly depends on an intimate give-and-take from a dedicated senior physician. "You need to find someone to be your mentor," says Adina Kalet, a family practitioner at New York's Gouverneur Hospital, who has written widely on mentoring. "Well, that's fine if there are people available, but there aren't." She says busy senior physicians are too preoccupied with nonteaching duties and interests. Yet studies in medicine, business, and elsewhere prove that "people who could identify individuals as mentors actually are more successful." Another internist commented that "role models are everywhere, but not mentors—not someone to interact with you, to guide you, to teach you the art and the morality of medicine." This is especially troubling as senior physicians fade away; those who can remember an era when mentoring was still the norm. Soon this older generation, coming of age in the forties and fifties alongside physicians brought up in the prewar preceptor system, will be gone, severing a critical link with one of Osler's generation's most important tenets.

This reminds me of something a medicine intern once told me, after trying to find someone to talk to about how to handle a difficult patient, a chronic drug abuser with swollen kidneys, who was demanding to be released from the hospital against medical advice. "In my vast experience of exactly one other patient like this," the intern said in a deeply frustrated voice, "I had no idea what to do. I felt like legally I had to let her go, so I did. But she was back a day later, in much worse shape." He said this had really bothered him—not because he didn't know what to do. He knew he had no choice but to let her go. The problem was the moral vacuum in which he was operating, and how important it was at that moment for a seasoned senior physician to reassure him that he had done all he could to help this woman. One wonders what William Osler would have said.

■

Of course, amidst all this physician grousing about the lack of sagacious overseers we should not lose sight of what this system can augur for patient care. As Rich Ferrara's experience suggests, an arrangement that depends too heavily on resident-based care can have a tragic downside.

There is also the matter of residents supervising residents. This was part of the problem in the Libby Zion case, where an R2 told an R1 to give an agitated Zion a small dose of Demerol, which he had seen administered in an oncology ward to stop patients on chemotherapy from shaking uncontrollably, a condition known as "rigors." As it turned out, Demerol is seldom used for someone in Zion's condition— something a senior attending almost certainly would have told the residents, had one been present. An attending also might have warned the residents that Demerol is potentially lethal when mixed with a medication Zion was taking at the time: Nardil, a powerful antidepressant. One theory about how Libby Zion died is that these two drugs interacted and killed her.

Wayne Osten, head of New York state's hospital investigations unit, told me about an error that he attributed to a system where the almost blind lead the blind. It occurred in October 1994 at Albany Medical Center in Albany, New York, when a senior resident told a PGY1 to order "TPN"—an intravenous form of nutrition—for a five-year-old patient. The PGY1 "had only done one of these before," Osten said, "written a TPN order, and he asked assistance from a senior resident." The senior told the PGY1 to check the bag of fluids used previously to see what mix of fluids to order. "The order called for dextrose, 50 percent dextrose solution to be added to the TPN," explained Osten. "He misinterpreted that and ordered dextrose 50 percent concentration of the whole TPN," when in fact 50 percent referred to the total calories the dextrose should contribute.

"The entire system," said Osten, "broke down because it went to the pharmacy. They didn't catch it, and they said after we interviewed them that it was the largest order of dextrose they had ever seen in a TPN order, but they didn't question it." The next day the same thing happened again with a new PGY1. "To his credit, he went to his senior resident and told him, 'I've never done this before,' so the senior resident says just repeat the order from the day before. So this five-year-old kid winds up going into a coma. Her glucose level was 2,000." A normal level is 65 to 115. "She recovered," said Osten, "but then died." They didn't perform an autopsy, he added, because she was terminal with cancer.

"This was a classic case of a PGY1 not having any experience," said Osten, a longtime investigator who advised the Bell Commission in 1987, and has checked up on thousands of adverse incidents in New York state. He added that this sort of thing can happen anywhere, even in a hospital like Albany, which "is a pretty good hospital, pretty responsive."

According to the state's official report on the incident, which cites a violation of New York's supervision laws, Albany Medical Center told investigators they "took immediate action to ensure that pediatric TPN orders are appropriately reviewed by a supervising resident or attending physician. In addition, the pharmacy will confirm orders in which the TPN components are outside ranges developed for the facility." In other words, the hospital promised investigators they would be more careful next time—and reorganized their system of TPN orders to the satisfaction of state investigators. Yet the possibility remains that a similar situation could happen again with another drug or treatment, either at this hospital or elsewhere; where residents don't know what they don't know.*

■

Bill Frishman was in trouble. Running late to his eighth-grade son's basketball game, he was going to catch hell with both his son and his wife. Rushing through the early evening traffic on the Bronx River Parkway toward his home in Scarsdale, this forty-eight-year-old cardiologist had been up since five A.M. and had just finished twelve hours presiding over a substantial medical fiefdom. The epitome of the "triple threat" attending, Frishman manages or co-

*I asked Albany Medical Center for a statement on this incident, but did not receive one after repeated attempts.

manages research grants totaling millions of dollars a year. He serves as the associate chairman of medicine at Bronx's Albert Einstein College of Medicine; is a member of an academic cardiology practice at Wyler Hospital, a division of Montfiore Medical Center, following some 2,000 research and private patients a year; is a full professor of medicine and epidemiology at Einstein—and, this month, is an attending physician for a team of two interns, two medical students, and one senior resident on the general medicine wards at the Bronx Municipal Hospital Center.

As headlights blazed past on the parkway, Frishman seemed remarkably energized given what he had accomplished that day— one that was not yet over, since after his son's game, he would retire to a second-floor study at home to read journals for an audio series he edits. Ironically, given his schedule, the series annotates important journal articles that doctors can listen to if they don't have time to read the journals themselves. Tomorrow morning, Frishman planned to rise at four or five o'clock to work on a paper he will submit to the *Journal of Circulation*, on left ventricular hypertrophy. "I also have some grant proposals to look over tonight," he said, shifting lanes in his sleek red Mitsubishi 2000—"My one indulgence," he says.

One would think it would be exhausting to be around Bill Frishman. But perhaps the most remarkable thing about this small man with wiry, wild gray hair, gray beard, and squared, silver-rimmed glasses, is his calm. As I followed him that day, he showed remarkable imperturbability as a whirlwind of activity swirled around him.

I soon discovered his secret, realizing that Frishman is a master delegator who leaves most of the details to others. The only time I saw him really hunker down was during a two-hour stint after lunch in one of his offices—he has at least three—when he churned out several letters, most of them dictated to a secretary in rapid-fire progression, and made calls. The rest of the day he attended meetings; and, because the Jacobi–Einstein campus is enormous, he did a lot of walking, going from one office or research area to another.

At first, all this walking seemed like a waste of time, until I saw that every few minutes he ran into a colleague with a question or concern. "A lot of the collaboration that goes on happens when you bump into each other," he said with a smile, looking a bit like a mad scientist with his unruly pile of curly hair and crisp white lab coat.

■

I met Bill Frishman that cool morning in January in the main lobby of Bronx Municipal—a sprawling complex of buildings in a leafy neighborhood on the northeast side of the Bronx, just north of what one attending here called "the frontier" of inner-city decay. Over-crowded with indigent patients, many of them recent immigrants, and chronically underfunded, Bronx Municipal looked a bit bedraggled, with old, worn furniture and carpeting, and walls of mustard-yellow glazed bricks set off by equally repulsive shades of beige and light gray latex. But the hospital was clean, and it provides good care.

Frishman greeted me warmly and beckoned me to follow as we headed toward his first stop for the day. On the way, he told me about his team of residents. "They are an interesting group," he said, waving his arms for emphasis, and standing so close to me that I could feel the warmth of his breath, a style of speaking he continued to use throughout the day. "A Pakistani resident that started [on the ward] yesterday. One intern from India, and a black woman, I don't know where she is from yet. And two third-year medical students: one is Taiwanese and the other is an American from India. It's an international group, and they just started yesterday on the wards. They presented their first cases to me yesterday."

Frishman said the team's load was very heavy at the moment. Two days earlier, they had admitted five patients, for a total of twenty-two under their care.

"Is that a lot?" I asked.

"For two interns, yes. People are usually very complicated. They'll come to a city hospital like this with multiple problems and are often very sick." He added that the team was on "long call" tonight, with the intern on call admitting patients all that day, and through the night until nine the next morning. (This is different from short call, where interns accept new patients only until nine P.M.) Interns are on "long call" every fourth night, and on "short call" every second night after long call. Because New York state by law limits residents' work hours to no more than twenty-four hours a day and an average of eighty hours a week, interns are supposed to go home early the next morning after long call.

Sometimes they don't, however. No intern I spoke with could remember a single overnight when they went home before noon the next day. One intern drew a chart for me of his last week, claiming he had worked some ninety-three hours. He said he seldom went home before ten or eleven at night on days he was not on call, and stayed until dinner time when he was postcall—for a total of thirty-six hours in a single shift. If he maintained this pace all month—which he expected to do—his hours would technically violate the law.

Frishman said he spends an average of two hours with the team during attending rounds, six days a week—commencing most days at ten A.M. He also drops by on some afternoons before heading home. Otherwise, Frishman kept to his routine of research, writing, seeing private patients, and walking the halls—reachable at all times by beeper for calls or questions. He admitted he was seldom contacted, however, telling me that interns tended to go first to their R2, the chief resident on their floor, or to the in-house attending who was, by law, always available in the emergency room.

I asked him if he should spend more time with his residents. Possibly, he said, though he insisted they had to learn how to "stand on their own," offering an example from the Disney movie *Bambi* of what he considered a perfect mentor/attending, trainee relationship.

"You remember that Bambi spends most of his time with his mother," said Frishman. "His father only shows up to help him when he is in trouble. The best example of that is at the end of the movie when there is the fire. Bambi is trying to escape and is panicking. It looks like the end when his father appears and shows him the direction to go and then leaves him again. So Bambi crosses the finish line himself with his father looking from afar. This means that when the residents fall we are there to help them up. When they are doing a good job we are there to complement and reinforce them. The mentor's job is partly to show the way, but to allow the individual to cross the finish line himself/herself, allowing each to stumble and pointing the way when necessary in the right direction."

"But what sort of stumbling is admissible," I asked, "and what is not? Is it ethical to purposely allow someone to possibly stumble when you are dealing with human subjects?"

"I think it is ethical in that people are being supervised. There is always someone above you to answer to. So I think that in most situations that minimizes the initial chance of harm."

"These patients on the ward, they're officially your patients, right?"

"They are my patients. If the residents make a mistake, I am technically responsible."

"Does that make you nervous?"

"Yeah, but that's why I tell them to call me. It's part of them learning to use their own judgment."

At Bronx Municipal, Frishman explained that they comply with the Bell Regulations governing supervision by assigning one attending to be in house every night for all eight medicine teams manning the wards and the ICUs. This supervisor is called the "405 Attending," after the numerical designation for this rule in the state code. There also is an attending in the E.R. "Years ago, when I was an intern, it was just the interns, on all night by themselves," said Frishman. "The intern was the first line of defense. That was a little too much to put on anybody. Besides, we made mistakes. And that's what the resident is there for. The intern explains what he wants to do and it may be completely wrong but at least there is somebody listening to say no, you should do it this way."

"But what if the R2 doesn't know? Or thinks he knows, but is wrong?"

"Hopefully, they'll call someone else who does know. That's what they're supposed to do."

■

After attending grand rounds between eight and nine A.M.—the topic was severe acidosis, a common malady among alcoholics—Frishman started his morning custom of promenading from one project site and office to another, winding his way through a labyrinth of buildings. In the hallways, he ran into several colleagues—including an epidemiologist with whom he is collaborating on a study, and a fourth-year medical student named Jeff Bernstein, who is helping Frishman on another research project. "I supervise about fifteen students in their senior year who have to write a senior thesis. Jeff is doing a project on EKG abnormalities in old people."

At 9:15, we visited one of his labs in the medical school, an NIH-sponsored project Frishman is co-managing as part of the national Women's Health Initiative. Funded by the NIH, Frishman explains that the Bronx is one of forty locales researching "all aspects of women's

health. Cancer. Nutrition. New cardiovascular drugs, lipid problems, high blood pressure." His specific task will be to follow 4,000
women for eleven years, testing what Frishman calls "the estrogen
hypothesis. Whether or not estrogen in postmenopausal women
will prolong life. Specifically by preventing coronary events, osteoporosis, memory deficits. It is the largest NIH trial ever done on this
subject." He introduced me to the nurse who oversees the project's drug
trials office at Wyler Hospital, and grimaced at his full in-box in a small
office. Next, we strolled over to the clinic to check Frishman's
schedule of private patient appointments for the next day.

■

At 10:15, Frishman ushered me up to 3 South, a busy public ward
with rooms holding four patients each, each one visible from the
hallway through large windows in the walls, meshed in wire safety
glass. Just beyond a busy nursing station Frishman pushes open a
door into 3 South's conference room—a small, stuffy room where
the heat was cranked up far too high. Everyone was perspiring. The
faces of the residents and medical students waiting for Frishman
were flushed.

With Frishman presiding at the head of the table, intern Fiona
Bayne, twenty-six, from Great Neck, New York, presented a case—a
thirty-seven-year-old man admitted because he was disoriented and
slurring his words, but he was not drunk or on drugs. Frishman
asked several questions about the family. He then digressed to tell the
team about cases of hereditary psychoses, which have been exten-
sively studied in twins. The residents enjoyed the digression—they
were *excited* by it, and eager to learn. Over the next hour and a half of
attending rounds, Frishman digressed several more times, on subjects
ranging from HMOs to Alzheimer's. At one point, he asked the
women on the team if they want to join his NIH estrogen study.
"Estrogens are, for women, clearly the elixir of youth," he pronounced with his endearing, mad scientist grin. "We think it prevents
heart attacks, probably because it prevents plaques from cracking"
and coming loose in chunks that can lodge in valves and vessels,
interfering with blood flows and precipitating strokes.

In between digressions, Fiona and other members of the team
presented other patients—an eighty-four-year-old man with a heart

problem who seemed to have pneumonia but might be septic ("Did you rule out meningitis?" he asked; they had, said Rajat Goel, the other intern); a twenty-eight-year-old male who overdosed on cocaine and was suffering from a pulmonary edema, and possibly tuberculosis; a forty-five-year-old man with emphysema; and an eighty-six-year-old woman who fell in her house and hit her head, possibly because of a stroke.

Despite his tangents, Frishman asked good questions. He motivated the team to learn. For instance, when the team presented the woman who fell, he asked: "Why do women get more fractures?"

"Osteoporosis," said one of the medical students.

"In fact most of the morbidity and mortality for very old women is from osteoporosis."

Later, during bedside rounds with the team, Frishman talked to this eighty-six-year-old woman and asked her several questions: How did she fall? Where was she when she fell? After she answered them all in a weak but clear voice, he turned to me as we left and said out of hearing from the team, "I think this woman just had a fall. I'm not going to tell the resident what to do, though. It's up to him."

"So you wouldn't have admitted the woman," I said.

"Yeah, because she just fell. She remembered what happened. I've seen people who faint and lose consciousness. She didn't. She remembers exactly what happened."

I asked why he didn't send her home, suggesting that she looked extremely uncomfortable in her hospital bed. I also remembered something Bertrand Bell had once told me, that a hospital is a place where bad things can happen, especially to old people, who are susceptible to catching viruses and often fail to thrive in unfamiliar places.

"It's not my call," said Frishman. "I leave that up to the resident."

After attending rounds ended at about noon, Frishman dove back into another day of chance encounters, conferences, and correspondence. First off, he met with medical students complaining about the restoration of "honors" as a grade—which they insisted was pushing an already intense and competitive program over the edge. Frishman later said he suspected the students' real problem was that some had barely missed getting honors.

Shuttling from office to office, Frishman then wrote letters and answered calls before dashing off to another meeting—a cardiology conference about using inotropic drugs to stimulate calcium receptors in the heart. He cut out early to return home, hoping to make it to his son's basketball game before it was over.

■

Exceptional, versatile, and empathetic, Bill Frishman comes as close as anyone to pulling off the old "triple threat." During a brief visit, I was unable to verify if his hands-off style with residents provided the most optimal care for his patients. I suspect, however, that the system as Bill Frishman has organized it works well enough most of the time, as it does in most hospitals—including Jim Stern's and Bill Kidd's.

Still, one wonders what would have happened if, for instance, an attending at Stern's hospital had been more involved in the case of Mary Allen, or if a senior supervisor had peeked in on the "bad boys" at about two-thirty A.M. during that hot July night. For that matter, was it right to allow a frail but reasonably healthy eighty-six-year-old woman to stay in Bronx Municipal, when she clearly wanted to go home—merely so that a team of residents could exercise judgment?

I was not with Frishman every minute of the day, but during the afternoon, I never saw him make contact again with the team on 3 South, though he said he might phone the senior resident to check in that evening. (He did, about ten o'clock, telling me later he did this "because the team was new.") "I'll be there again at ten tomorrow for attending rounds," he added, talking up close to my face again and waving his hands. "That's all I'm technically supposed to do, unless I get called in."

I know for a fact that the residents did not telephone Bill Frishman that night, because I returned to the hospital and stayed with them for most of Fiona Bayne's call. According to the interns, the attending would be one of the last people they would contact. "I would first find one of the in-house senior residents," said Bayne, "or ask someone down in the E.R. if I had a question. Otherwise, I'm on my own, I guess."

■

Not every attending shares Frishman's rapport with residents or has his natural gift for teaching, even if he spends only a small part of his time on the wards with the house staff. Indeed, yet another drawback in the current system of teaching is that it depends heavily on the personality and style of each attending. To some extent, this cannot be avoided in any teaching system that relies on individuals, though residencies seem particularly susceptible to the whims of seniors and supervisors.

"Some attendings," noted Benjamin Frain, one of the interns on Jim Stern's team, "find it a chore and leave us hanging, and then just show up to go on a quick attending rounds. They act very busy, like this is taking time away from something important. Then they just sign off on our notes, because they legally have to, and they're gone, and we hardly ever see them."

Even worse are attendings who tutor by intimidation and fear. Stories abound about infamous senior doctors in years past who yelled and screamed insults at residents, and constantly grilled them on arcana. One surgeon in Texas is said to have drawn a chalk line just inside the entrance to the surgical wing of his hospital, telling residents he would work them so hard they would not have time to ever cross that line. Another attending in North Carolina reportedly told his interns three rules: (1) Never use a dog if you can get a house officer; (2) Bleed him until he faints; and (3) Do it again.

Usually, the intimidation is more subtle, though every bit as real, as an anesthesiology resident found out during one of her first cases in the O.R. Describing her attending for the operation as "a very strict, difficult man to get along with," she says he asked her the day before the case to read up on a narcotic called dilaudid, to determine the dose for the patient and have it ready for the procedure the next day.

That night, however, she worked so late in the O.R. that the library was closed by the time she finished. When she couldn't find anything about the dosage elsewhere, she decided to ask a fellow, saying she didn't dare ask the attending. The fellow told her to infuse 0.2 mg per kilo, and to redose it every two hours. "This was a very bright guy who had finished his residency and was doing his fellowship, and I trusted him. So I opened about ten vials of dilaudid and diluted them up in one large syringe." As it turned out, the concentration was ten times more potent than it should have been. The resident's attending, however, started the operation without asking her anything about the drug. He just "began pushing the syringe on the patient."

It turned out the dose was supposed to be only .02 mg per kilo. Because of the error, the patient remained intubated for several hours after the operation. "Luckily there was no long-term problem from it," said the resident, "but there easily could have been if it had been a more dangerous drug. The patient also happened to be a really big guy, over six foot and muscular, so he could absorb more of the drug than most people. I should have double-checked with the attending that morning, but I was sufficiently intimidated at that early stage in my residency and I was trying to prove myself."

During a vascular surgery operation, I saw an attending turn around and scream at the top of his lungs at an intern who had come into the O.R. to impart an urgent message from another attending— that one of his patients had been sent to the ICU because of an infection. "I don't want to be disturbed in the middle of a procedure to hear shit like this!" screamed the attending. "You are fucking out of line, coming in here to my O.R. and telling me this shit!"

Of course, business, law, and certainly journalism also endure their share of bastards who torture underlings. But again: in these other professions, working under a browbeating boss is dangerous only to that underling's peace of mind, unlike medicine, where teaching and managing by fear can result in harm to patients.

■

Given the tremendous weight of tradition, economics, and convenience underpinning the chief resident arrangement—and, in some cases, the almost religious adherence to the dogma of the see one, do one, teach one—it takes tremendous effort and courage for an attending to buck the system. In all the time I spent following residents, I met only a handful of senior physicians who attempted to put teaching first and refused to endorse the notion that attendings should remain mostly in the background. One of these was a thirty-two-year-old primary care physician named Jennifer Jeremiah, who spends most of her year as a clinician associated with Rhode Island Hospital. Teaching, however, is her first passion, so she spends three months of every year attending. "This is where my interests lie," she says. "I love to teach."

Unlike most attendings, however, Jeremiah cuts back her other activities substantially so she can spend more time with her residents. "I set aside the day to do this. I'm probably losing money by spending so much time teaching. But I believe this is the way it should be, because for most doctors, it's not a high priority."

Following her around during a two-day stint, I saw her spend several hours a day on the wards, not interfering or doing the thinking for her charges but really *teaching* them. "I believe in asking a lot of questions, and in didactics where it makes sense," she told her team on their first day together. She also announced that they were her priority this month. "I have cut back my office practice to about half-speed, so I can be here for you guys," she said to them, handing out several phone numbers. "I will be more angry if you don't ask than if you do." Later she told me that with a greenhorn team like this one—this was their first month on the wards—she would rather have them ask questions than try to do everything on their own.

For instance, later that morning, when one of the interns admitted that she did not know how to properly percuss (tap with her fingers) an abdomen to figure out the size of the liver, Jeremiah—a thin, attractive, professional-looking woman with shoulder-length hair and a single strand of pearls around her neck—marched down to the patient in question and gave the intern a fifteen-minute lesson.

Jeremiah could be tough. When one intern grew flustered before her first patient presentation, constantly glancing down at note-cards, Jeremiah told her gently but firmly to pocket the cards and tell her about the patient from memory. After a moment of panic, the intern took a deep breath and recited the information. Later, Jeremiah told me she could sense the intern knew her stuff but had never been pushed to organize it in the sort of public manner a physician must be able to do. "So much about teaching, and supervision, has to do with the individual residents," said Jeremiah, in a statement Osler would have agreed with. "People have different skills. People have different strengths.

"It's important to find attendings who are effective teachers," she adds, "who love teaching. There should be a large group of them. We should have doctors who are teachers first and foremost. But there are not, and this is a very bad thing."

■

In the end, claims Bertrand Bell, it's the patients who matter most. "They're the ones paying the bills," he says, and who expect to receive optimal care from a fully qualified physician. "The contract," he says, "is between the patient and the attending, not between the patient and the resident. People aren't coming to this hospital to be taken care of by an intern five months out of medical school." Bell said he could remember in the sixties when it became standard practice for residents to write orders for patients, rather than attendings. "I told them to forget it. These were my patients, and I would only let residents write orders for them when I knew I could trust them. These patients are depending on me.

"Being a doctor is the best thing in the world," says Bell. "It's fun. It's challenging. It's a privilege. You can do good. But you have to remember what the purpose for all of this is. It's to heal people. To take care of them while we educate new doctors. That's why we wanted to have people always on duty to ask questions to—a collegial system of people working together to make sure people learn something, but not at the expense of patients."

CHAPTER 5

Balm of Hurt Minds

Most of us are scared we'll get tired and do something wrong. It's very hard to work and think you might get so tired you'll hurt someone.

Internal medicine resident, PGY2

Why am I so angry?" asks a frustrated Ben Rollins. "Because I need a cardiology consult, and I can't find one." Two patients had crashed in the last two hours, he says; another had just landed on the floor with "about eight things wrong with him," from throat and colon cancer to emphysema and vascular disease. "I arrived today and suddenly had nine patients," he fumes. "I just started this rotation, and I don't know these people." Almost as an afterthought, the twenty-eight-year-old intern adds: "I'm exausted. I was here until eleven-thirty last night, post call," meaning he been going full bore for three days with just eight hours rest.

I'm following the tall, lanky Rollins as he strides down a corridor. He's holding a two-inch-wide strip of paper seven or eight feet long, the end trailing along behind him and dragging on the floor. Rollins stares at the EKG blips on the tape, but he is so exhausted the information doesn't register. "This is too disorganized," he mumbles, his eyes swollen and bloodshot. His long, dirty-blond hair juts out at odd angles. It's greasy, as if he hadn't washed it in days. "I've got too much to do. This isn't me. This isn't my personality."

Rollins's ordeal began the previous Sunday, when he was on call in the hospital's bone marrow transplant unit. "I was up all night Sunday," he says, logging almost forty hours straight without sleep on Sunday and Monday. He returned at 8 A.M. this morning, Tuesday, launching into a new rotation on the oncology ward. Now it was late afternoon, and Rollins would be here until almost midnight, when he would go home to rest a few hours before plunging into another call day tomorrow. Starting again at eight, he would work all day, all night, and all the next day until at least dinner time, for a staggering total of 91 hours out of a possible 108 hours over a five-day period. Rollins said the back-to-back calls was a scheduling error, though when I asked if was going to complain, he said "no," that in his program, interns were expected to handle anything. "You've got to be tough," he later told me.

Back with Rollins the next night (Wednesday night) at nine-thirty, I find him in even worse shape. "This is a nightmare," he says, plodding with a tired man's gait through a crowded ward of patients in chemotherapy, radiation treatment, and end-stage cancer, with several being tended at a level approaching intensive care. At the nurses desk, banks of monitors beep and flash vital signs. Phones ring and buzzers sound as nurses, techs, and aides come and go in flashes of white and blue.

"Dr. Rollins," says a nurse, "the woman in 416 still wants you. She has this rash on her hand." Rollins doesn't acknowledge her as he folds up another EKG he has been reading, carefully creasing the edges several times. Only after they are sharp as a blade does he turn to look for 416's chart, rummaging through a waist-high cart of shelves mounted on wheels. "Yeah, well, shit, wouldn't you know it. Somebody's got her chart." He slams down one of the blue folders onto the stack and looks up at me, realizing I am watching. "You know, I hate having you here right now," he says. I offer to leave, but he says no. "I'm just usually not this disorganized," he says, his voice suddenly apologetic. "I'm not usually this upset. Really."

As I followed Rollins around for the next hour and a half, I kept waiting for someone to tell him to go home—a nurse, the cardiologist who finally showed up to read the EKG, or another intern who

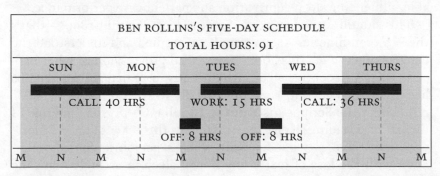

BEN ROLLINS'S FIVE-DAY SCHEDULE
TOTAL HOURS: 91

SUN	MON	TUES	WED	THURS

CALL: 40 HRS   WORK: 15 HRS   CALL: 36 HRS

OFF: 8 HRS   OFF: 8 HRS

M   N   M   N   M   N   M   N   M   N   M

M = MIDNIGHT   N = NOON

brought up a meatball sandwich, Rollins's dinner, from a local deli. I asked the head nurse if she thought Rollins looked tired. "Yes, he does," she said. "This happens all the time. It's not healthy. We help them get through it, especially when they're just starting the rotation." I mentioned that he had gotten almost no sleep in the past four days. Wasn't that dangerous?

"We'll keep an eye on him," she said.

"When would someone be so tired they would be sent home?"

"I've never heard of that happening," she said. "I know of some who have gone home because they were sick. But they have to be practically dead. There's this thing about being tough with them."

■

It's hardly a revelation that medical residents are frequently exhausted. For years, reformers have been calling for a reduction in residents' hours, insisting that whatever benefits might come from following patients for the classic thirty-six-hour shift—whether it happens every other night, every third night, or every fourth—is more than outweighed by the dangers of severe sleep deprivation. This is more true than ever as young physicians try to absorb a crush of new technology and information, and when trainees are directly supervised by senior residents sometimes as sleep deprived as they are. At least one study suggests that even twenty-four-hour shifts may be pushing it. Conducted by a prominent hospital in the East, this unpublished internal analysis of their own house staff concluded that seventeen hours, and the number of successive days of more than seventeen hours at work, "is the most important variable influencing sleep deprivation and patient care performance."

This should surprise no one. Since at least the mid-1890s—that's the *eighteen*-nineties—scientists have studied and understood the dangers of sleep deprivation. "The lawful progression of what happens when you deprive sleep either totally or in little bits and drabs has been worked out," claims Merrill Mitler, director of sleep research at the Scripps Institute in La Jolla, California, and one of the nation's leading sleep experts. He says this "lawful progression" is as inevitable as what happens when a person is denied water. Even with the loss of just a few hours' sleep in a single night, he contends, "reaction time slows, ability to respond to new information is compromised," and the potential for errors increases greatly. Getting less than optimum sleep night after night can also lead to chronic sleep debt—a condition Mitler and other experts say can impact performance even if a person has had a good sleep the night before. "Ultimately," Mitler says, "in experimental animals if you deprive them of sleep long enough the animal dies."

Studies measuring the detrimental impact of fatigue on everything from small muscle coordination to complex decision making have persuaded officials in government and private industry to restrict on-duty hours of airline pilots, railroad engineers, bridge officers on ships, nuclear power plant operators, and factory laborers. Late last year, the Federal Aviation Administration, citing extensive data blaming fatigue on airline crashes, announced it will seek to cut the maximum hours a commercial airline pilot can be on duty from sixteen to fourteen hours, and to increase rest periods between shifts from a minimum of eight to ten hours. This follows the enactment of an FAA rule requiring that pilots take naps in the cockpit on trans-Pacific flights—a policy approved despite considerable opposition by airlines—because studies have overwhelmingly proven that naps reduce instances of pilots falling asleep at the controls. In the Persian Gulf War, the U.S. Army likewise ordered combat officers to get at least eight hours of sleep in every twenty-four, after extensive research demonstrated "sleep deprivation causes leaders to . . . make mistakes and decisions which cause the death of . . . their units."

Investigators have blamed several recent airline crashes and train wrecks on fatigued pilots and operators. According to the U.S. Department of Transportation, sleep deprivation causes one-third of all truck fatalities and over 56,000 auto accidents a year. Examiners have also blamed fatigue at least in part for the wreck of the *Exxon Valdez* and the near meltdown of reactor number three at Three Mile Island in 1979—accidents that occurred in the wee hours of the morning, when experts say the body's levels of alertness are at their lowest ebb, and the potential for drowsiness is at its greatest.

Over the past decade, researchers from Harvard University to the University of California at Davis, and from the University of Florida to Westminster Medical School in London have been amassing data on residents themselves—long a neglected area of study—strapping portable EKGs onto trainees' chests, videotaping them performing surgery, tracking their brain waves, and monitoring their eyeball movements at rest. Researchers have concluded that overnight shifts induce fatigue severe enough to impair a resident's logical reasoning, cognitive skills, creative thinking, and fine motor coordination.

Critics of these studies insist residents can overcome even severe fatigue by sheer willpower. Residents also say the terror of erring acts like a powerful jolt of caffeine. "You push yourself," said one PGY3, "and the adrenaline just kicks in, and you're okay."

Mitler agrees that physical movement can override fatigue—up to a point. "A basketball player playing basketball who's sleep deprived may do rather well," he says, "but a bookkeeper may not"—or a resident sitting and writing orders, catching up on notes, or trying to concentrate on a tedious task, such as inserting an arterial line, or holding a clamp in surgery. Fear and adrenaline, however, typically last no more than fifteen or twenty minutes before fatigue returns, he says. Mitler also cautions that a sleep-deprived person may plunge into action with the vigor and determination of someone fully awake, but frequently ends up following a strategy that may be flawed by sleep deprivation. "The effects of sleep deprivation are not professionally dependent," says Mitler. "You can't learn to do good when you're sleepy. What you learn to do is move around a lot and avoid tasks you're vulnerable at." It is also a symptom of sleep deprivation, says Mitler, that the sufferer does not realize how badly he or she is impaired.

■

Of course, most of us don't need stacks of alpha and beta brain wave charts or the Pentagon to convince us we need a good night's sleep, something Shakespeare long ago called the "balm of hurt minds." Nor does anyone who has had to stay up overnight and work the next day, or slogged through 80- to 100-hour weeks, need to be told by Ph.D.'s they do not function at their best. But most of us are not physicians, who as a group continue to deny the logic of history, science, and common sense, every evening of every week, conducting an ongoing experiment on thousands of young physicians such as Ben Rollins to see just how little sleep they can endure without faltering.

"It is rather incredible that things as important as human lives are being taken care of by people who are dead tired," says former surgeon and outcomes researcher Lucian Leape of Harvard, "working overtime and late at night. We wouldn't do that with most things in life. Most jobs in the world we don't do that. They don't want tired people running their assembly lines, yet we still do it in hospitals."

A few superhuman residents emerge unscathed, surviving with little effort on a few hours of sleep caught here and there. (I have not actually met anyone like this, though I am assured they exist.) And there are those who have runs of luck where they can get barely enough sleep—three or four hours on a call night, say, and more on nights in between. Yet if the studies and experts are correct, most will find themselves compromised as weeks of too little sleep pile up, a few devastatingly so.

Some residents react to extreme weariness with anger—like Ben Rollins. Others grow irritated. "It's hard to be pleasant right now," Bill Kidd told me twenty-two hours into his trauma shift. "I feel like biting heads off." Later, Kidd said he was so bleary-eyed at one point that he lost track of which patient in trauma was which. I asked if he was ever beat enough to stop and summon backup. "No," he exclaimed in his ironic voice, "are you kidding?" Still others respond with an exaggerated machismo, or with a stoicism that attempts to deny even the possibility of fatigue—such as the PGY2 in Boston who contracted hepatitis and hooked himself up to an I.V. pump attached to a portable pole. With antibiotics and fluids dripping into veins, he persisted in treating patients and performing his usual duties for two or three days, until his chief finally made him go home.

One intern told me he was feeling "numb" after putting in some thirty hours with only one hour of sleep. "I'm in something of a fog," he said, after I asked him for his home address and he could not remember it. Still working five hours later I watched him draw blood from a near-comatose patient. Jabbing at the vessel, he missed and poked a hole in the woman's arm. When she moaned, he said in an aggravated voice: "I know, dear, life's a bitch all over." Three hours later, as he was desperate to leave, a nurse asked him to draw blood from yet another a patient, a non-physician "scut" job he said he should not have to do. Angrily jabbing the unconscious patient's arm, he drew out the blood, capped the glass tube, and furiously ripped off his gloves. "Now, how are they going to hurt me next?" he asked. "Or can I go home now?"

In a 1994 documentary titled *Bad Medicine?* by three students at the Columbia School of Journalism in New York—one of them is the wife of a surgical resident—a resident recounts the time another trainee in her program passed out in the operating room from exhaustion. She woke up in a hospital bed hooked to monitors, admitted as a patient. Another told about falling asleep during surgery and dropping to the floor, where he faked a convulsion to avoid a reprimand. One seemingly unflappable chief resident, known for his calm and humor, told me he responds to stress and weariness by holding it in—and has the ulcers to prove it.

For Frank Ingulli, a third-year medical student, fatigue proved fatal as he drove home one night at one forty-five. He had just finished a grueling stint in a surgical clerkship at New York's New Rochelle Hospital Medical Center, and accidentally turned onto an exit ramp on Interstate 95. Hit head-on as he motored south on the northbound side of the highway, he was rushed back to the same operating room he had just left. Surgeons he had been assisting a couple of hours earlier tried desperately to save him but failed. State police investigators blamed the accident on fatigue.

In New England, another exhausted trainee, a resident, went home post call and self-administered a dose of insulin for his diabetes. He then fell asleep without eating—and was dead within a few hours from insulin shock.

■

A few weary-to-the-bone residents develop more than just bad attitudes, when fatigue combines with stress to push them over the edge into bouts with clinical depression, alcohol, and drug abuse—and, in extreme cases, suicide. Precise numbers are hard to come by. Most studies about severe physician impairment use either "soft" data—surveys and the like—or extrapolate from small groups of subjects that may or may not be relevant to the almost 100,000 residents and fellows, and 650,000 total physicians in the United States.

But even these sketchy figures indicate that the human toll of stress and fatigue among physicians is alarming. According to the research, a physician is up to three times more likely to commit suicide than someone in the general population, though Harvard sleep researcher Gary Richardson has told me that he believes suicide among residents is not appreciably higher than it is for young lawyers and others in high-pressure professions. Other research suggests that physicians abuse alcohol and certain drugs more, and possibly a great deal more, than the general population; that interns have a one in three chance of suffering from "frequent or severe episodes of emotional distress"; and that a higher than average percentage of doctors find themselves in dysfunctional marriages and relationships. In 1991, AMA researchers determined after an extensive survey that 71.6 percent of residents had observed colleagues, including attendings and nurses, impaired while on duty. The most frequent impairment was fatigue (58 percent); others included emotional problems (39 percent), incompetence (39 percent), alcohol consumption while on the job (16 percent), and drug abuse (5 percent). Dr. DeWitt C. Baldwin, Jr., then the AMA's director of medical education, presented these figures at a residency forum during the organization's annual meeting near its Chicago headquarters. He pronounced residency impairment a "serious crisis."

Most residents and young physicians I spoke with knew of somebody in their medical school or residency who had attempted to kill themselves, some successfully. One OB–GYN resident said two people had already taken their own lives in her hospital that year. "I guess suicides are common here," she said. Another young doctor, a chief resident, said he knew of five suicides in his programs since he started training: two in his midwestern medical school, one in Texas during his residency, and two so far among the hospitals affiliated with his current program during the nine months he had been chief. Anxious to put the best face on these tragedies, he said: "Well, the person in Texas was a drug addict. She was an anesthesiologist who overdosed." One of the more recent deaths, he said, was related to "severe depression"—as if the stress of training had nothing to do with pushing them over the edge.

On the plus side, many programs in recent years have not only recognized the reality of impairment, they also have organized counseling sessions, spouse-support groups, and the like, indicating a willingness among some educators to be open and frank about depression and other problems, and to listen without criticizing or exacting punishment. But one psychiatrist who counsels depressed rcsidents told me the macho imperative to hold it in and ignore it remains potent. "Depression among doctors is viewed as a weakness," she said. "The danger is to laugh it off, to deny the stress. Residents are at high risk."

■

Back on Four South, after eating his sandwich and swigging a Coke, Ben Rollins went to see the woman with the rash on her hand in 416. Stepping into the private room was a strange transition from the crowded, glaringly lit corridor. A long-term victim of cancer, this patient had brought from home a lamp with a pastel yellow shade and low-wattage bulb, a tape recorder playing soothing New Age music, and a small library of books and puzzles. A hand-lettered poster encouraged "mom" to get well. The steady beep of a heart monitor and several I.V. pumps in the corner were the only obvious reminders of where we were.

The woman was thin but still energetic, wearing a brown wig and makeup. She sat up in bed and asked Rollins's name, adding with a sigh that she wished they would stop changing doctors on her. "I was just getting used to the last one," she said. Clasping her hand, Rollins asked how badly it hurt, though it was obvious her rash—a drug reaction from chemotherapy—was not why the woman had asked to see him. Speaking calmly, she announced that she had decided against the experimental treatment the oncologists had proposed as a last-ditch effort to save her. "I'm at peace with this decision," she said softly, holding Rollins's hand in hers, the music swelling like an ocean wave. Her eyes glistened with tears. "When I came in here, I thought I would try everything. I'm concerned about—dying. But I know this treatment will be painful, and it may kill me before my cancer does. I want to enjoy the time I have left. I love my family. I don't want to miss this time."

"We'll do whatever you ask," said Rollins, trying to sound empathetic, but not entirely managing to suppress the edge in his voice.

"But what do *you* think?" she asked of the proposed treatment, as if she wasn't entirely sure. Rollins was interrupted by his beeper before he could answer. "Got to go now," he said tersely, promising to return later.

Closing her door, Rollins pivoted toward me with a pained

expression and blurted out: "That's *exactly* what I mean. That woman has decided to die, and I don't have time to talk to her about it. Even if I did, I wouldn't know what to tell her. I haven't had time to read up on this treatment. I don't know much about onc[ology]. I'm dealing with things I don't know about, like this drug. By the end of the month, I will have learned a lot. But I need to know it *now*." I thought he might break down and cry, but he didn't.

I remembered a young physician on the West Coast who, exhausted, had to inform a patient he had AIDS. "I took about three minutes. I told him, checked it off my list, and went on to something else. It was a few minutes before I realized what I had done." He said he had to step into a supply room so no one would see him sobbing. "I had become a monster," he said.

Back at the station, a nurse tells Rollins she can't locate a patient whose chemotherapy treatment has wiped out his white blood cells, leaving his immune system so weak that he could easily catch a serious infection. "He is roaming around the hospital," says Rollins, who explains that it is his responsibility to keep a close watch on this man. "I'm feeling guilty, because he could die just like that." Rollins's beeper chimes again. Checking the number, he explains it's the E.R. "Another admission," he groans. A second nurse informs Rollins that a walk-in admission has arrived and is waiting in the lounge with his family. The first nurse says a patient needs more morphine, and Rollins asks her how much he should give, telling me that these things aren't taught. "You just learn them, usually from the nurses," he says. Uncapping a pen to sign the order, he contemplates the rack of overflowing medical charts and the banks of monitors. "*Beeeeeeep!*" brays the pager. "This is a nightmare," he mutters. "I'm having too much going on to handle this."

■

As far as I know, Ben Rollins's fatigue resulted in nothing worse that night than an unhealthy bedside manner. Given the statistics, and the extent of his sleep deprivation, he was perhaps lucky. For instance, in 1991, a study published in the *Journal of the American Medical Association* reported that 41 percent of residents polled listed fatigue as a major cause of errors—with 51 percent reporting mistakes due to "too many other tasks," and 54 percent because they "did not know information they should have known." In almost one-third of the cases, the residents said that their errors resulted in the death of the patient. Again, questionnaires are no substitute for solid clinical data, though these findings suggest the potential scope of the problem.

So do a seemingly endless profusion of anecdotes. For instance, *Time* magazine reported that in California in 1990 a resident fell asleep while sewing up a woman's uterus—and toppled over onto the patient. "In another California case," reported *Time*, "a sleepy resident forgot to order a diabetic patient's nightly insulin shot and instead prescribed another medication. The man went into a coma."

Among the residents I interviewed, an OB–GYN resident told me she once fell asleep while performing a cesarean, scalpel in hand. (She woke up instantly and finished the operation.) Another said she was so tired one night she ordered a potentially fatal dose of Ativan, fortunately caught by a senior resident. Likewise, many of the misadventures cited in previous chapters—including some of those committed by residents in New York and investigated by the state's department of health—transpired many hours into an on-call shift.

I've followed more than one resident who erred when reasonably well rested, though most problems occurred either deep into the night, or post call. Indeed, residents nearly always blamed fatigue or ignorance, or both, for their mishaps, insisting that if they had been more awake, they might not have missed the diagnosis, or the proper dosage. "Ask any resident if they have the potential to make more mistakes when they're tired," asked an intern at a busy hospital in New England, "and most, if they are honest, will say yes." Another said: "Most of us are afraid we might get tired and make a mistake. The potential is always there."

At the very least, maintained the Boston OB–GYN, an exhausted resident is less enthusiastic about being thorough. "You try to get out of work," she said. "You are lazier because you are exhausted. The way I treat my patients, I'm not as good to them. People suffer, and maybe the public doesn't realize it, but they do." She said the worst thing was to be called by the emergency room at four or five A.M., with a patient who is ill but not critically. "You try to get out of it," she said. "You try to say, 'Well, just send them to the clinic tomorrow,' when really the person is worried enough about themselves to come into the hospital, sit in the emergency room for three hours, to tell you their personal problem about some delicate GYN thing at two A.M.. And then you turn around [and tell them to go home], just because you're too tired after twenty-four hours. It's not the best thing to do."

"House officers can be ruthless in preserving the precious hour or two of sleep they may be able to take while on call," wrote Timothy McCall in the *New England Journal of Medicine*. "Rather than replace a patient's intravenous line in the middle of the night, they routinely substitute intramuscular medications, ignoring the question of patient discomfort and the possibility of more erratic absorption of the drug."

Several nurses I talked to confirmed that a tired resident tends to be less responsive than one well rested. "Fatigue does affect them," observed a nurse in a large southern hospital. "They respond more slowly. They need more time to think. Sometimes they lose it, they have to go compose themselves." Another said: "You may call an intern in the middle of the night, and say I need a night order for somebody. Maybe a potassium level's low, and they'll say, 'Okay, why don't you do this, why don't you do that,' but they won't come and write the order. And it will slip, because they are so exhausted."

Compassion also suffers as fatigued and stressed residents lose their capacity to empathize and sometimes even hate their patients for forcing them to stay awake. "One night when I was really exhausted," said a surgical resident in Seattle, "this patient came in by ambulance with a heart attack. It was four in the morning, and I'd been up since eight the morning before, and up late working the night before that. They gave her streptokinase, a clot dissolver, in the ambulance,* to break up a clot in her coronary artery. This medicine can cause a person's heart to become very unstable. They can arrest and code multiple times. I remember being so tired and pissed off that I didn't know how to manage this patient. I wasn't getting any supervision, and I remember thinking, God, I wish this woman would just die. She kept coding, and it was like she was torturing me. I took it very personally. This was a horrible experience for me. I still feel guilty. She later turned out to be one of the nicest patients I've ever had. She kept thanking me for saving her life. Tears were running down her cheeks."

*Streptokinase in this case was given by EMTs under the direction of a physician in contact with them by radio.

Psychiatrists have written about physicians actually hating patients who are abusive, unresponsive, or extremely difficult to manage—an attitude compounded by fatigue. One young attending told me that even when she is well rested, "not all of my patients are lovable. Some yell at you, try to physically attack you." A surgical intern added that it was "hard to empathize with a patient who is spitting in my face."

Even when patients are not difficult, residents' daily jargon occasionally bristles with idioms denigrating their charges. Two researchers at the University of California at Berkeley, Victoria George and Alan Dundes, listed in a study some of the terms used by residents: "turkey," "crock," "trainwreck," "lizard," and "reeker." There also are "noncitizens"—drug addicts, bums, alcoholics, and the homeless, which are distinguished from "citizens"—the clean, the receptive, and the insured. "Is he a citizen?" I hear weary residents ask when called with an admission from the E.R., watching as their attitudes sour when the answer is no. "It's another thirty-something I.V. drug abuser noncitizen who's going to make my life miserable," said one resident, "and keep me up half the night."

No term is more prosaic, or bitter, than GOMER—Get Out of My Emergency Room—immortalized in the satirical novel *The House of God*, by Samuel Shem, loosely based on his internship in the early 1970s. "Gomers are human beings who have lost what goes into being human beings," explains Shem's character known as The Fat Man, the novel's embodiment of the brilliant but cynical second-year resident who guides the interns on his team through their first year in the *House.* "They want to die," he continues, "we will not let them. We're cruel to the gomers, by saving them. . . . They hurt us, we hurt them." The notorious term "Gomer" is passé these days, but the sentiment, at times, remains.

■

Educators seem aware of resident fatigue. Yet most insist it doesn't affect patient care. "No one can find data that fatigued house officers kill people," contends Frank Spencer, former president of the American College of Surgeons and a professor of surgery at New York University Hospital. He spoke these words during a 1991 debate on residency issues at the summer meeting of the AMA, in Chicago. A traditionalist who believes residents are far too coddled today, Spencer admits that fatigue is a problem, but as a detriment to education, not because it harms patients. Yet he defends the every-other-night call system as the only real way to teach surgery, insisting that slipups are impossible because attendings monitor residents, tired or awake, too closely. "They are supervised," he said. "They have colleagues. They are cross-checked. All your professional life you work when you're ill, when you're tired. The same cross checks occur for the house staff. So the fatigue thing is not true."

At the other end of the spectrum are educators who fret constantly about their residents' ordeal, with a few conducting what amounts to their own personal experiments in sleep deprivation, spending many extra hours a week counseling trainees in distress. Even in the most resident-friendly programs, though, educators continue to sanction eighty-, ninety-, and one-hundred-hour weeks.

But why go through all this in the first place? What is the urgent, compelling need that justifies putting residents and patients through an experience that should be tough and challenging, but is often miserable and potentially dangerous?

The reason most often given is "continuity of care," an educational imperative that insists a young physician must follow patients as long as possible, to study them for subtle changes as treatments are tried and disease takes its course. "There is no substitute for the resident watching patients closely overnight," said one medical chief.

Few would argue with this in theory. But even assuming residents can handle the long hours, there is another problem—residents are seldom *with* patients at night. More often, they are jotting copious notes and organizing orders (like Jim Stern), chasing down lab results and X rays, or waiting for the E.R. to send up admissions. Patients also don't always oblige the thirty-six-hour shift by arriving in the first hour or two, to allow for maximum continuity of learning. Most appear in the late afternoon and evening, or overnight. Nor do most patients require minute-by-minute care. Even if they do, residents are frequently too busy, or overwhelmed with a ward full of sick patients and scut, to glean a meaningful educational experience from every charge.

And what about the 4,000 nonteaching hospitals in the United States? They cover patients exclusively with attendings and nonphysician staff, who are not expected to work anything approaching thirty-six hours. Presumably, these charges do not suffer from a lack of continuity of care—or from the practice of passing on patients among several physicians as they change shifts.

"There is no scientific support," wrote Timothy McCall in his *New England Journal of Medicine* article, for the claim "that long hours improve the experience of learning during the residency. . . . Nor are there data to support the contention that the quality of care is improved. That a discipline so dedicated to scientific proof would base its whole training system on untested assumptions is curious."

In 1991, educators at the Veterans Affairs Medical Center in Minneapolis, after switching their residents to a night float system, found that lessening hours *improved* some measures of care—and may have saved the hospital money. Patients' length of stay dropped from 10.9 days before to 9.3 days after, according to this study, and laboratory tests ordered for each patient fell from twenty-four to nineteen. Residents also made fewer medication errors, dropping from almost seventeen per one-hundred patients discharged to twelve.

Harvard sleep researcher Gary Richardson dismisses the notion that residents must stay up for reasons of continuity of care as "hogwash." A vigorous immersion in medicine is important, he says, but not to the extent that trainees are grossly deprived of sleep. Richardson says the real impetus behind the hours and overnights is economic—the fact that residents save hospitals and attendings time and money by manning the wards overnight and on weekends; and by freeing attendings to see private patients, teach, and conduct research.

Indeed, the historic underpinnings of physicians' long hours have less to do with watching the progression of disease than with the rise of the modern hospital, which coincided with around-the-clock treatments—and the need for somebody to care for patients at all times. In the early days, however, most everyone understood this arrangement was more a convenience for senior doctors than an educational experience. Today, this has been largely forgotten as long hours spent in the hospital are considered crucial not only because of continuity of care, but also as proof of one's commitment to medicine. Of course, some say that patients like having their doctors always there—which may be true, though patients I talked to told me they would rather have a well-rested doctor than one who was always available, if that meant he or she was fatigued.

■

There is a residency director in Washington, D.C., who reportedly greets his new interns each year by telling them: "You will be working at times for twenty or thirty hours without sleep; it will be hard but you will be better physicians for it." Another director warns prospective interns that they will compress forty-eight hours of tasks into twenty-four hours, because this is the only way to fully embrace medicine.

This Puritan work ethic run amok has engendered strange theories among physicians that they can tolerate fatigue and stress to a far greater extent than others. "The public," said one chief resident, "has a perception that we work too hard. But we self-select. We try very hard here to get people who are excellent." John Potts, chief of medicine at Massachusetts General, told me he is not convinced fatigue is a problem. "Nor is the house staff," he said, according to a poll that asked his residents if they ever felt impaired by fatigue.

Obviously, physicians must be able to function at times when weary. But there are limits. "The medical community," says Merrill Mitler, "is saying that somehow the laws of physiology apply to everyone else, but not to them. They say, 'But we know we can stay up, because we have done it.' This is like doctors at the turn of century refusing to wear sterile gloves when they operated because they had operated many times without a sterile field and had their patients do fine."

Researchers blinded by the belief they are genetically superior when it comes to sleep have even promulgated questionable studies to support their contention. When I spoke with Frank Spencer, he cited a 1988 study on drowsiness in residents, published in the *Journal of the American Medical Association*, which concludes that residents can handle an every-other-night call schedule without getting unduly fatigued. In the study, researchers tested surgical residents for impairment after serving a thirty-six-hour shift, reporting in *JAMA* that the difference between the on-call surgeons and the controls was negligible. "Sleep deprivation," they asserted, "did not affect overall cognitive or motor performance."

Critics at the time claimed the study was seriously flawed, however. "The residents," wrote Harvard's Timothy McCall in a letter to *JAMA*, "served as their own controls: the study compared them when sleep deprived—after a night on call—with when rested, after a night off. The authors assumed that residents who slept the previous nights were rested, but this is hardly a safe assumption." Noting that sleep deprivation can last longer than twenty-four hours, McCall claims the results were faulty because the control group was most likely chronically sleep deprived from their ongoing call schedule. Yet I still hear surgeons mention this study as proof they are different from pilots, combat officers, and even their colleagues in general medicine and other nonsurgical specialties.

But let's say it is true, that doctors *are* self-selected. They're motivated. They're committed. They're physiologically adapted to require less shut-eye. Even so, at some point they *must* sleep—even if they can tolerate twenty-four hours, thirty-six hours, three days, or five weeks. More importantly, they must stop and live, if only to better understand their patients, and themselves. "I'm something of an addict for working too hard," said William Hazel, an orthopedic surgeon practicing in Virginia. I spoke with him soon after he finished his residency at the Mayo Clinic in Minnesota. "I try to adjust more to my values, to lighten up, to spend time with my kids, because I don't want them to live like this. But I have a hard time. This is the way I was trained. This is what we were told we had to do, and now I know it is wrong."

■

At 12:01 A.M. on July 1, 1989, a new era dawned in the United States for residency work hours—or so it seemed at the time. This was when the Bell Regulations went into effect in New York State. Also called the Libby Zion Rules, they became law five years after the death of this eighteen-year-old woman at New York Hospital, and four years after the grand jury looking into Zion's death lambasted the residency system in New York State. Recommended by then state Health Commissioner David Axelrod, and approved by the state Hospital Review and Planning Council, the laws forbid residency programs in all 114 teaching hospitals in New York—the largest concentration in any single state—to work their residents more than an average of eighty hours a week, or more than twenty-four hours in a single shift.

Initially, the council mandated that the state, Medicare, Medicaid, and private insurers pay for additional hospital staff to compensate for work previously performed by residents working over eighty hours. In 1990, Harvard researcher Kenneth Thorpe postulated that this would cost hospitals $358 million a year; what insurers and the state have actually handed over is closer to $200 million a year. These amounts acknowledge just how much labor beyond the eighty-hour barrier was extracted from residents in New York prior to 1989—and is still expected in many states without hours limits.

Hailed by reformers as the first major wave of what was expected to be laws passed in several more states, the highly visible process that ushered in the Bell Regulations also contributed to moves by many programs across the country to voluntarily reform themselves before government legislators did it for them. In 1991, the major accreditation body for residency programs, the Accreditation Council of Graduate Medical Education (ACGME), provisionally enacted new service hour guidelines for most residency programs. The AMA did the same soon after. By 1992, all the organizations governing specialties followed suit—including surgical boards whose membership initially rejected even the most minimal reforms. They acquiesced when key legislators in California and Massachusetts threatened to support government-imposed mandates without them.

Mostly, the changes codified modest reforms already in place, including a switch from the traditional every other night on call to every third night. There were, and are, many exceptions to this. Even today, some surgery programs persist in an every-other-night call schedule, in violation of the new rules. Meanwhile, most internal medicine programs have switched to every fourth night, though a few stay every third. Innovative programs in the immediate post–Bell Regulations era also introduced "night floats"—residents who oversee wards late at night, so the on-call residents can theoretically rest or get caught up on their admissions. Yet another reform is programs that place caps on the number of patients a single resident will admit when on call. These "caps" range from five to nine patients, though in most hospitals I visited, residents are sometimes forced to exceed their limit if patient volume is heavy, usually because there is no real backup system.

Most educators breathed a sigh of relief when legislation limiting residency hours died or failed to pass in Massachusetts, California, and elsewhere—and then was pushed aside soon after by the larger health care reform debate launched by President Bill Clinton in 1993–94. Antiregulation fever sweeping the country in the mid-nineties also stymied efforts to reform by government fiat, a not entirely unwelcome situation, given that it will always be more effective to persuade physicians and educators, rather than force them into innovations they believe are wrong. To date, no other state has enacted Bell-style laws.

∎

I wish I could report that the voluntary guidelines, reforms, and regulations have succeeded; that all residents in the United States are well rested and no longer stressed, depressed, and overburdened; and that patients are no longer at risk from resident fatigue. In some programs, this may be true. But in most of those I'm familiar with, reforms have only slightly improved the lot of residents, while patient outcomes, inasmuch as they have been accurately measured, remain unaffected.

Keep in mind that since 1989, the fund of medical knowledge and new technologies have continued their wondrous and relentless expansion. Also consider that patients who wind up in hospitals are sicker than ever, and staying in-house for shorter periods, particularly in an era of managed care. There also is less sleep and down time when on call than, say, twenty years ago, because there is more to do. As I suggested earlier, all this adds to an ever greater intensity per hour facing residents, even as educators insist trainees are toiling fewer hours than in the past. Or are they? Studies claim residents spend an average of seventy to seventy-five hours in the hospital a week—with interns and surgeons working up to ninety and one hundred hours a week. But these numbers include low-labor intensive disciplines such as child psychiatry—which often has an every eighth- or ninth-night call. (In a survey taken at an East Coast Hospital, child psychiatry residents and fellows worked 43.8 hours a week, followed by dermatologists at 48.4 hours; and nuclear medicine at 55.5 hours.) Eliminate these specialties, and averages begin to climb. Many of the surveys also make no distinction between intensive rotations and, say, electives, where there is little or no call, which further lowers the averages.

When I followed medicine interns on the wards and in intensive care—the most rigorous rotations of all—I counted an average of about 90 hours a week, with some bumping up to the occasional 100-plus-hour week. A very few, like Ben Rollins, pushed over the 130-hour threshold in a single week, out of a possible 168 hours. This compares to 110 to 117 hours a week under the old system of every other night on call, with a day off every other weekend. (This assumes residents in Bob Nye's generation, and those just after, never slept while on call; in fact, Nye and others say they slept several hours most nights.) Surgical residents I tracked often logged 100 to 110-hour weeks. A few specialties tallied even more, with the East Coast hospital survey claiming an incredible 138 hours in the hospital a week for cardiothoracic surgery fellows.

Most programs are expanding the amount of time spent on outpatient rotations, particularly for primary care specialists, though these less strenuous stints through daytime clinics and outpatient O.R.s are often combined with evening and all-night shifts in the emergency room. Residents on primary care rotations are also called in as backup on the wards and ICUs for residents who stay home sick or have taken a maternity leave.

Typically, residents I followed caught some shut-eye during overnights in the hospital. Bedding down in tiny on-call rooms for anywhere from a few minutes to a few hours, they took catnaps tending to last from two to four hours. Even this brief respite was almost always disrupted, however, with pages from nurses asking permission to administer drugs, or with updates on patients. "Even when you sleep," observed a medicine resident in New England, "it's interrupted constantly. It's not satisfying sleep." The longest stretch I witnessed during my twenty resident-nights was five hours—which was violated only once, when a nurse called about a dosage of Demerol. My intern said this was a world-record snooze for her, ten months into her internship. As I have noted before, even on noncall nights residents frequently stay very late—sometimes past midnight for days on end—with a starting time for surgeons as early as 5:30 A.M.

Obviously, medicine residents racking up an average of 90 or 95 hours is preferable to 100-plus-hour weeks in the past, and 100-plus hours for surgeons is an improvement over 110 to 115 hours. However, in talking to department chairmen, chiefs of service, and even a few residency directors, I was surprised to learn that they believed their trainees were in-house more like seventy or eighty hours a week. Consider the chairman of surgery I met at a prominent hospital in Washington, D.C. With an intern I was following sitting with me in his office, I asked him how many hours his residents worked. "Far fewer than they used to," he claimed, estimating they averaged no more than eighty hours a week. The intern, an outgoing Persian-American woman with long black hair, smiled broadly when he said this. "That's not right?" asked the chairman, looking at her quizzically.

"It's more like a 110 hours a week," she said, "or 115."

"Is that true?" he said, genuinely surprised. "I had no idea."

Other chiefs and senior attendings stridently maintain that young doctors not only work fewer hours, but also have made such an issue of their own lifestyle needs that it has lessened their commitment to patients. One attending in New York City, who trained in the early seventies, told me the Bell Rules had produced physicians with a "time clock mentality," who don't always know their patients intimately because they are not in the hospital enough. "What you miss these days is the sense of continuity we had," he said. "It used to be, somebody would grab you and say, 'What was Smith's blood sugar?' and we would tell them, because we would know everything about him, as if someone were to ask about your child, at what age they first sat up. That's how well you knew these things. Now they don't."

"So you are saying that if you ask one of your residents a patient's blood sugar," I said, "and this was important to know, they might not know it?"

"That's right," he said. "Somebody knows on the team, but not always the intern, or the resident who took the test. You see, it may be over twenty-four hours, and they don't know because their shift is over. When they're off, they're off now, whereas we just knew."

This belief was reflected in a survey done of attendings and residents at the Albert Einstein School of Medicine in the Bronx, which reported that while "residents agreed that the regulations diminished their fatigue, had no impact on their ability to observe the full impact of interventions on patients, and resulted in better patient care, attendings were uncertain or disagreed." Attendings "agreed" on the survey, however, that the Bell Regulations "had caused a shift-work mentality among residents." This prompted me to ask virtually every resident I spoke with in New York if he or she could reel off the latest vitals on their critically ill patients. All of them could. One PGY2, suturing a patient at three A.M. in a busy E.R., became incensed that an attending would say such a thing. "I am deeply offended by the idea that I would not be there for my patients, and not know everything there is to know about them."

"I personally, and so do many of my peers, find it insulting that some would think we would walk away from a patient without providing continuity of care," said California resident Rebecca Patchin at a 1991 meeting of the AMA. Patchin was then a senior officer in the AMA's Residency Physician Section. Pointing out that the critical issue is less one of continuity of care than learning how to pass on patients at the end of a shift, she noted that "at some point in our lives as physicians, we'll need to turn over patients to our colleagues, whether that's after six hours, or ten weeks." Even under the old system, she added, this imperative was largely ignored, and remains poorly taught—despite the fact physicians spend their entire careers passing on patients. "As a professional and as a resident I need to learn how to find out about my patients in a safe way for the patient," she said, "and in a manner in which my colleagues can properly manage that patient when I am not there."

■

Unfortunately, the news from New York State is not much better, despite the Bell Regulations being in force since 1989. While educators disagree on the ultimate success or failure of the law, critics contend that some programs are ignoring the rules, a few blatantly. Even at Bronx Municipal Hospital and Jacobi Medical Center, where Bertrand Bell still teaches and attends, interns say they often stay until evening or later, ordering tests, scribbling notes, and treating patients.

"We certainly don't schedule people for more than eighty hours a week," said Dr. B. Robert Meyer, director of general internal medicine at Jacobi, who has been a strong advocate of the Bell rules. "But these people are conscientious, and can't always wrap things up after eighty hours. It happens."

In fact, among the scattering of residents I interviewed and followed in New York, nearly all acknowledged they routinely labor beyond the eighty-hour average. Surgery programs, which won a last-minute exemption from the eighty-hour week when they threatened to challenge the rules in court, can legally put in the hours they always have, though surgeons are supposed to rest whenever possible, and to document it. Many do not, however.

One resident in New York City told me his program—a surgical subspecialty not exempted from the eighty-hour-a-week law—routinely faked schedules. "We write up the schedules that say we're in compliance," he said, "but we continue to do a traditional every-third-night schedule. You go in, say, on Monday morning, you work Monday night, you work all day Tuesday. You might get off at ten or eleven Tuesday night. Then you start again at 5:30 the next morning. They just tell Albany everybody leaves after twenty-four hours." In reality, he sometimes clocks forty-hour shifts on call. According to a 1994 report on residency code violations written by Mark Green, Public Advocate for the City of New York, state health investigators have cited numerous programs around the state for failing to obey Bell provisions on hours. Citing an exhaustive list of violations, Mark Green's report concluded that "New York City resident hours routinely exceed the Bell Regulations' eighty-hour work-week limit." The report failed to emphasize that most violations are eventually corrected to the state's satisfaction—though the point is that the infractions have occurred at all, particularly at such a high rate.

Operating on a shoestring budget, state monitors can only visit each hospital in the state about once every five years.* For instance, in 1993, Wayne Osten's investigators visited twelve hospitals according to state reports. All but one had at least a single program failing to comply, including two that were not obeying the limits on hours—North Central Bronx Hospital and King's County Hospital. (The others violated the rules on supervision and or the credentialing of procedures.) In 1992, seven out of twelve hospitals investigated transgressed in at least one department. In 1991, the number was fifteen out of twenty-four hospitals.

*The state by law is supposed to investigate hospitals every three years. Because of budget cuts, the state health department has scaled back to visiting each hospital every five years. In 1995, Governor George Pataki proposed eliminating investigations altogether as a cost-saving measure.

For example, in 1992, St. Luke's/Roosevelt Hospital in New York City was cited because "Residents were scheduled and did work more than twenty-four consecutive hours," and for other hours violations. Included in a long list of specifics was the following:

SURGERY:
- On-call residents in Surgery were not generally resting at night, and/or their rest was interrupted frequently, and/or they were on call more often than every third night, and/or the on-call night duty was not followed by at least a 16-hour non-working period.
- According to [name deleted], PGY1, admitting residents at St. Luke's get 2 to 4 hours sleep when on call and work a regular day post call.

PEDIATRICS:
- 1/15/92, 8 A.M.–5 P.M. regular work, then on call at 6 P.M. to 8 A.M. on 1/16. Then 1/16 from 1–4 P.M. in Pediatric Continuity Clinic (once per month).

According to the law, programs found in violation are placed on probation, and have from one to three years to correct the deficiency. If after this time the program is still determined to be in violation, the state can either shut down the program—something they have never done—or levy fines that average $2,000 per violation. In the case of St. Luke's, neither happened, since the hospital was able to correct its hours deficiency to the state's satisfaction.

Green's report offers one explanation for the seemingly widespread noncompliance, quoting medical educators fiercely opposed to restricting hours. "A physician in the pediatrics department of Mount Sinai Hospital we interviewed," writes Green, "believes so strongly that the regulations interfere with patient care, that he admitted his department had opted to give itself three hours beyond the twenty-four-hour shift, in open violation of the law. 'Let them put us in jail,' he said. 'They should accept the realities of this world and Dr. Bell should be sent somewhere else.'" Another critic, Thomas Gouge, director of the surgical residency program at New York University Medical Center, is quoted in the film *Bad Medicine?* blasting the Bell dictums as producing less than committed doctors. "If you can't stand the heat," he says, "get out of the kitchen."

"The bitterness and viciousness of some opponents still shocks me," responds Bertrand Bell. "You would think our commission had radically altered life as we know it. All we did was say to ease off a bit. It's not that much to ask."

Other reform-minded educators agree, though few I spoke with believe the Bell provisions have been entirely successful, if only because they still ignite such rancor and turmoil. "It might have worked better if this was done more gradually," said one attending in the Bronx, who supports the rules. "We tried to shove this thing down people's throats, people who have the power to resist. I mean, what is the state going to do, shut down New York Hospital because residents are working eighty-one hours instead of eighty? Or Columbia-Presbyterian?"

■

One of the most contentious issues raised by the Bell laws has been their impact on patient care, a question that lingers unanswered because no one has conducted comprehensive studies. In one of the few attempts to assess the new code, researchers perused state outcomes data and concluded that patients tended by residents during the first year of the Bell era had suffered a slightly higher rate of minor medical complications than they had during the final year of the old regime. In all other categories—mortality, transfers to intensive care units, and length of stay—the outcomes were unchanged. A similar study conducted at the same time at Columbia-Presbyterian likewise found no change in patient outcomes. This prompted its authors to conclude that the Bell Rules had failed, though another explanation might be that the system was too new to have made any great impression.

Only one aspect of the New York regulations on hours is truly unambiguous: resident satisfaction. Every survey reports that residents who feel their programs are complying believe they are better rested. Almost everyone notes that the rules have considerably boosted morale, compared to earlier years. Residents, at least, believe they are doing better at taking care of patients than in the pre-Bell days.

Bertrand Bell himself, sitting in his office at Bronx Municipal surrounded by photographs of friends, family, and important political allies of the past (like many liberals in New York, he is out in the cold during the Pataki years), is unabashedly proud of his efforts, despite the controversy. Ensconced behind a cluttered desk not far from the hospital's emergency room, where he began his own career forty years ago as an intern, Bell confesses to a certain sadness at the sustained resistance of his colleagues.

"The intention of the commission was for people to come up with new ways of teaching postgraduate medical education," he says. "None of us ever dreamed you would have programs continuing to simply keep going on the old call system, trying to fit it into the new laws. Of course, you're going to fail. The old system depended on residents running things twenty-four hours a day. If you don't change that fundamental fact, you're either going to have to greatly increase the number of residents, or break the rules."

■

By now, as the hours debate continues year after year, the issue seems frankly more absurd than ever. One must remember that even the reformers are advocating hours anyone outside of medicine would consider outrageous. Indeed, the scale of expectations is way off, given that no other industry would be screaming to be allowed to work *only* eighty hours a week, and *only* twenty-four hours at a time.

On average, Americans toil just under forty hours a week, for a total of 1,951 hours a year—second only to Japan, whose workers put in 2,155 hours a year. (Germans spend about 1,603 hours a year on the job.) By contrast, residents working "just" eighty hours a week, with a three-week vacation, spend *3,920 hours* in the hospital—twice the national work average. Those grinding out ninety-hour weeks amass an incredible 4,410 hours. There is a word this reminds me of, *mumpsimus,* defined as "a traditional custom or protocol obstinately adhered to however unreasonable it may be."

In the end, the hours issue boils down to a simple fact, that this is something physicians can control when caring for patients, which means they have an obligation to thoroughly understand its impact, and to know without a doubt that what they are doing is safe. At the very least, medical science should be rushing to study physician fatigue, on the off chance that the weight of sleep science outside of medicine might also hold true for doctors. Someone also should be looking seriously into how many hours, and what mix of sleep, naps, uninterrupted sleep, and time away from the hospital is optimal, just as the FAA and NASA have intensively studied this question for pilots, and spun off scientifically valid numbers that even airlines have been forced to acknowledge, despite a powerful incentive for them to avoid spending money on extra crews and on berths in cockpits for napping pilots.

Meanwhile, residents like Ben Rollins labor on in a senseless test of endurance, caught in a limbo between tradition and common sense.

In a letter published in *Texas Medicine,* a physician in Houston summed up the frustration of many doctors sick and tired about the issue of residency hours. "Will the controversy be put to rest?" he asked. The answer, I believe, is that it will not as long as physicians condone what the rest of us consider highly abnormal conduct, particularly when the justifications are at best controversial, and at worst dangerously mistaken.

CHAPTER 6

Scut and the 20% Solution

The training of a resident physician has been called one of the last great sweatshops in America.

Laurie McKeown, M.D., chairperson,
AMA Resident Physician Section, 1991

I punch the start button on my Casio stopwatch and watch the numbers tick off as Cindy Williams, a short, dark-haired medicine intern with thick glasses and a quick wit, launches into what we dub "the great X ray quest."

On the tenth floor medicine ward, she grabs an x-ray order written earlier for a certain Mrs. Morro. "This is a fifty-seven-year-old woman with various things wrong with her," observes Dr. Williams, "including possible pneumonia. Hence, a chest X ray, ordered this morning, and taken. But so far, no film has shown up." Williams says she needs the X ray to strategize a plan of action for Mrs. Morro. "This is typical," she vents. "I wait, I call rays, I wait, and it doesn't come up. So I have to leave the floor and get it myself."

Usually, says Williams, she "burns up" about twenty minutes chasing down a film, because it involves a trek to the x-ray records room, located in another department, on another floor. Williams says she also can fritter away another five to fifteen minutes tracking down a radiology attending or fellow to help her read it.

Because the elevators are intolerably slow in this forty-five-year-old building, Williams shoves open the fire door beside the service elevators at 01:43:36 seconds into our search. She bounds down the steps, her white floor-length coat billowing up behind her. A steady traffic of mostly residents runs up and down the bare, musty concrete stairwell. "If we had to depend on the elevators," said one medicine intern, "half our patients would die."

03:17:44 We arrive at the basement level. Williams bursts out into a dimly lit corridor and strides down it like she's late to her own wedding. I ask if she feels frustrated. "Murderous is the word I'd use," she grumbles, adding that she "really hates" to leave the floor for something like this. "People have patients crash when they leave. It hasn't happened to me, but it's like bad luck. Leave the floor, boom. Crash."

05:08:37 Blasting through another fire door, Williams sprints up another flight of dim concrete stairs, rushing upward to the third floor of another tower in the hospital complex. Down another corridor, two lefts, and we're standing at a window counter, like in a post office. Inside we can see several rows of gray metal shelves stuffed with oversized manila file folders holding x-ray films, marked by multicolored tabs—oranges, blues, yellows, greens.

05:47:12 Williams gives the clerk her patient's name and a date. "That's the patient's mother's birthdate," she explains. "That's what they use here. Everyone else in the hospital uses medical record numbers. Except for X ray. I have no idea why."

06:12:46 We wait while the attendant hunts for the film. "This won't be typical if they can find it," says Williams. "I'll be very upset if this is my first good experience with X rays."

"You mean you usually don't find it?"

"Never."

"Where is it when you eventually find it?"

"It could be anywhere. X-ray heaven. Usually it's back here somewhere, but there's no one here to get it, or it's not where it's supposed to be."

08:23:03 The X ray is not filed where it is supposed to be. The attendant's baby-step pace visibly annoys Williams. She looks ready to explode. Finally, the clerk reaches the files and randomly thumbs through several hundred folders.

10:25:27 Still waiting.

12:58:34 The attendant discovers the X ray. "It's a world record," says Williams.

But the attendant says she can't hand over the film. "We haven't done the paperwork yet," she says. Williams looks like she might go supernova. In a measured, firm voice she says: "Look, I need to look at this *now*." She offers a compromise, suggesting that the clerk give her the film to look at, while the clerk keeps the manila "jacket," which has all its identifying markings on it, to finish the paperwork. When the clerk reluctantly agrees, Williams snatches the film and rushes down the hall, with me in tow.

14:13:57 It's a short walk to the x-ray room, where the walls are wallpapered with light boards. There's no "rays" fellow or attending in sight, but Williams's chief resident happens to be there looking at an MRI.

16:23:12 The chief helps read Williams's film. She says that Mrs. Morro "probably" has pneumonia. "You could go with that for now if you have to," she says, pondering the poor-quality film. "But I'd confirm it with rays"—i.e., a radiologist. I ask Williams if I can press "stop" on my watch. "Not yet," she said. "We still don't have a clear reading. . . ."

■

Some ten hours into a thirty-hour shift, this is an incredible waste of time for Dr. Cindy Williams, who will repeat this once again late that night, and several times during her next rotation on the public wards. Virtually every time I followed residents, I watched them struggle to shore up the sometimes gaping holes in basic hospital services, even at some of America's most prestigious facilities.

At one top hospital I followed an intern who drew blood nine times during a single on-call shift. "It involves finding a form," said another intern, "finding supplies, and finding a vein. You then have to walk the samples to the lab." He had twelve patients of his own that day, and that night cross-covered twenty more for his team. Drawing blood can take between twenty and thirty minutes each time, for a total of some three to four hours on that particular night. Another resident claimed she started nineteen I.V.'s in a single call shift—a total of four or five hours; fully one-eighth of her thirty-six-hour shift. "It just makes you lose more sleep," she said.

One intern I shadowed overnight on the East Coast doubled as a transport orderly, several times pushing patients on gurneys to x-ray rooms and labs for tests. He wasn't officially required to do this, he said, but if he didn't, and waited for the hospital escort service, he was afraid his patients might suffer. "Escort service here is the Achilles' heel of the residency," he said with an edge in his voice. "I escort patients all the time. Fifteen minutes here, fifteen minutes there." He and some of the other residents complained about this to their chief resident and chief of service. "They told me I'm getting a chance to connect with the patient," he said. "That's bullshit. Most of the time they're comatose."

It doesn't seem like a lot to ask in academic centers with budgets in the hundreds of millions of dollars to provide basic backup support for young physicians manning the front lines of patient care, required to toil eighty- to hundred-hour weeks for a salary that often pays less than minimum wage. Even worse are affiliated teaching hospitals who have no costly academic or research complexes to maintain, and often profit the most from inexpensive labor. Some hospitals have attempted to improve things by hiring nurse-clerks to route resident orders, and teams to draw cultures and start I.V.'s. But year after year hospitals continue to use residents (and the occasional attending) as backstops for chronically understaffed ancillary services.

This reminds me of a scene in *The House of God*, where the main character, an intern named Roy, is stumbling around on his first day feeling frightened and overwhelmed. Then he spends a few minutes with a family that gushes with gratitude over the fact he is their brother's doctor. "I was moved. I was a doctor. For the first time that day, I felt excited, proud." The euphoria lasts but a moment, however, as Roy is inundated by a crush of lab tests, bowel runs,[*] and grunt work. He tracks down his R2, The Fat Man, and tells him, "I don't get it . . . This isn't medicine, this isn't what I signed up for. Not writing orders for cleanouts for the bowel run."

■

Originally a Norwegian word meaning the "short erect tail of a rabbit," *scut* in recent years has been seized by physicians as their own. I can find no published use of the word prior to the early 1980s, though older physicians insist it has been underground slang for considerably longer. For residents, the term usually refers to tasks ranging from starting I.V.'s and filing routine lab orders to finding clean sheets for the on-call room—tasks that seldom require

---

[*]A "bowel run" is part of a series of gastrointestinal tests that include an upper GI series, barium enema, liver scan, and so forth. In Shem's hospital, residents and/or nurses are required to "clean out" the bowel before a "bowel run" with a series of enemas and cathartics.

four years of college and four more years of medical school to master. For others, *scut* is defined as any onerous or repetitive task, such as writing discharge summaries, some of which only an M.D. can do. For our purposes, I'll defer to a recent study out of UCLA, which defines scut as "all work performed in the treatment of patients that could otherwise be carried out by ancillary or paraprofessional personnel (e.g., blood drawing and patient transport)."

Educators I spoke with estimate their residents devote 20 percent to 30 percent of their time to scut. One department chairman told me his residents did 20 percent "noneducational" and an additional 20 percent "drudgery." Not surprisingly, residents agreed they spent at least 20 percent of their time on scut, with some claiming as much as 70 percent. The UCLA study found that four teams of surgical residents, tallying a mean of ninety-eight hours a week, devoted 21 percent of their time to "scut." Put another way, the average resident slogs through the equivalent of two to two-and-a-half months a year on scut.

Obviously, this extra 20 percent exacerbates the long hours of residency. It's often the difference between getting enough sleep, seeing one's family, eating regular meals—and, possibly, between coping and depression, or worse. It also suggests that residents like Ben Rollins, Jim Stern, and Rich Ferrara sometimes stay up and lose sleep not for educational purposes but to perform tasks that a clerk or orderly could do.

■

Educators swear they abhor scut. "The drudgery work is anathema to me, and we try to minimize it" says Jim Stern's chief of medicine, a tall, earnest man who has been known to refer to his trainees as his "children." He adds that if money for ancillary care could be increased, "we could shorten some of the hours that are not really related at all to medical judgment."

By my count, at least four hours of Jim Stern's day was consumed by scut (which he confirmed)—13 percent of his thirty-one hours on call. Had he been able to use this time to sleep, Stern might have logged four to five hours in his bunk, not the fifty-five minutes he actually got. When I raised these observations with Stern's chief, he frowned and said that paying for more hands to back up residents was not popular at a time when hospitals were cutting costs. Blaming a lack of public support, not hospital policy, he insisted: "We try to minimize it within the limits that we have to work with, and that's why I'm so angry about the lack of appreciation."

An assistant chief of surgery in this same hospital said essentially the same thing. "You have to do what you can to protect residents," he said, "to protect their well-being as much as possible. You should be thinking in terms of relieving them from other things so they aren't losing sleep because of scut work that somebody else could do."

Yet both of these men have a great deal of control over their departments' budgets, submitting priorities that range from faculty salaries and how many defibrillators are needed on their units to whether or not more nurses must draw blood. "If the chiefs wanted to keep their blood-drawing teams to help out the residents," said John Schibler, chief financial officer of Rhode Island Hospital, which recently had pruned blood-drawing teams to save money, "we would certainly reevaluate it." (Schibler explained that the cuts come in the face of dropping revenues from managed care insurers and from cuts in Medicare and Medicaid.) In this case, however, at least one chief at Rhode Island told me he was unaware of the cutbacks, because none of his residents had complained. This was despite an ACGME report in 1994 that criticized the hospital for not providing "appropriate" blood-drawing services at night—a matter they say was reported to them by residents. Schibler said he would investigate the blood drawing policy and correct it, if necessary.

■

Beyond pure scut are the many hours swallowed up by residents writing notes on patients. Almost always, they write them by hand; few hospitals I've visited have invested in computers for resident chart entries. (In part, this is because physicians have not pushed this issue, with older doctors trained before the computer age preferring pen and paper for chart work.) Work areas remain remarkably low-tech as we approach the year 2000. Most have, at best, a computer or two to transmit lab data, though a few hospitals are putting on line more sophisticated systems.

For 15 1/2 hours, Jim Stern churned out notes and placed orders.

This was fully half his thirty-one-hour shift—and noticeably longer than most residents I observed, particularly surgeons, who are infamous for scribbling notes that medicine residents insist are *too* brief. No nonsurgical resident I followed, however, set aside fewer than eight hours writing notes on a call night.

These late-night marathons of felt tip and paper bely the image conjured when some educators defend long, overnight hours in terms of continuity of care. Indeed, one has a mental picture of a resident hovering over a critically ill charge, adjusting I.V. flows, ordering and receiving tests as Mrs. Smith or baby Jane waxes and wanes. Nearly every older physician I met has a story about pulling up a chair to watch over Mrs. So-and-so, to make sure she survived her operation, or that the antibiotics had kicked in. The reality, though, is often very different. Every night I stayed up with residents, other than in the E.R. and surgery, they sat up much of the night writing chart notes—long, detailed accounts of what transpired during the previous day, including test results and analysis, suspected diagnoses, and plans. "By writing the note even the senior physician is forced to examine any new information that has come in about that patient and to gather his thoughts," explained Jim Stern's chief of service.

They are also important to the chain of command, since at some point senior residents and attendings will scan the notes, and either sign on their approval, or suggest changes. Hopefully, at this point, errors are caught—such as the time when the surgical resident sent home a little girl with a urinary complaint, only to have an attending read his notes and call the girl back for an emergency appendectomy.

But if residents really need this kind of time to catch up and sort out their thoughts—and an educational and legal obligation to record certain information in the chart every day—then why are they doing it at two A.M., four A.M., and six A.M.? Particularly on those nights when patients are stable and sleeping, and interns have admitted all the patients they are likely to get. As the debate rages over continuity of care, with some educators maintaining that trainees must stay up all night to watch the course of illness as it progresses, they should try staying up all night with their house staff. They would probably find that residents are frequently up scribbling notes and attending to scut, not watching disease unfold. In the Libby Zion case, for instance, the intern involved was not pulled away by a floor of crashing patients. Nor was she sleeping as nurses repeatedly informed her of Zion's deteriorating condition. She mostly sat quietly on another floor, staying up all night to compose notes and to organize orders—she also had one admission, and spent some time tending to other patients' routine needs—even as Zion's temperature hit 108 degrees and the intern heard a code, Zion's code, announced on an overhead.

"Sometimes, interns obsess with notes," opines a chief resident in another hospital. "To be frank, these residents find it easier to write notes than to deal with patients directly, especially interns who have been students all of their lives, and are more comfortable thinking and writing and analyzing tests. You also get the medical school mentality of staying up all night to study, something that only hurts *you* if you get tired. Here, it may hurt a patient if you're too tired because you stayed up all night writing notes no one will ever read."

When I went to talk to Jim Stern's chief resident, he broke down for me how many notes interns create each year in his hospital. He said they average fifteen to twenty progress notes each night on call—about one-hundred nights a year. "At the end of one year of internship," he said, "you have written somewhere in the neighborhood of 1,500 to 2,000 progress notes" while on call—in addition to those notes written on days when a resident is not on call. When I asked if this was necessary, he said no. "After you've written probably the first two or three hundred, you don't get much out of the last 1,700. To tell you the truth, they are not learning much out of writing their last several hundred."

If this is true, then once again we have a situation where the system seems absurdly excessive as residents lose sleep performing a function that ceases to be educational after three or four months. Why? Either because they think they have to—in which case they should be given time to articulate their observations at a more reasonable hour—or simply because *someone* has to produce the notes for bureaucratic and legal reasons. Either reason makes little sense as one sits up watching an intern scratch away in the still of the night.

■

Recently, some hospitals have not only eased scut by hiring new blood-drawing and I.V. teams, they've also added nurse/clerks to coordinate resident orders. A few have reorganized the physical layout of their facilities to avoid Cindy Williams's sixteen-minute search for an X ray several floors and a tower away. For instance, they've built small x-ray units, pharmacy dispensing stations, and labs for routine tests on each ward or patient floor, or every two or three floors. A surgical resident in Stern's hospital told me that since blood teams came on line earlier that year, he hadn't drawn a sample in two months. "Here we have available to us all these services," he said, "blood drawing, an electro crew to take EKGs, things that residents had to do until recently."

Other departments in Stern's hospital are not so lucky, offering blood teams and clerks only during the day, and at specified times. Cindy Williams's hospital provides blood-drawing teams only three times a day. Likewise, John Stobo at Hopkins told me three years ago about plans to build x-ray units and mini-labs on each ward. These remain on the drawing board, where they will most likely linger in an era of managed care, when many teaching hospitals are barely staying in the black, and some are dropping below the bottom line.

Every chief of service I spoke with seemed sincere in his desire to rid the resident world of scut, and to ease the burden for his trainees, yet the scut persists. According to one department chairman in a New York City hospital, it would cost about $200,000 to eliminate scut for every ten of his surgical residents. Let's compare that to the price of, say, a second, third, or fourth MRI* in a hospital. With a price tag of one million dollars, an MRI equals the cost of ancillary services for fifty residents—two-thirds of the residents in this chairman's program. But an MRI rakes in $500 to $1,000 for the hospital every time an image is taken. In a matter of months, the machine can pay for itself. Spending a million dollars to hire more ancillary personnel to protect residents would *cost* a million dollars, and not earn the hospital a dime.

When I posed this notion of MRIs versus scut reduction to John Stobo at Johns Hopkins, he was intrigued by the comparison, but said, "Unfortunately, hospitals and doctors don't think that way."

■

If scut is so abhorrent, and possibly hazardous in that it con-

*Magnetic Resonating Imager.

tributes to stress and fatigue, why does it continue? One answer lies in a cardiac operating room where I observed for an afternoon a couple of years ago.

The patient was a fifty-seven-year-old man—I'll call him Mr. Jacobs—lying anesthetized under gauzy green blankets. In a sterile field, his heart and lungs lay exposed and immobilized deep inside the open cavity of his chest. Surgeons were rerouting the plumbing of this two-pack-a-day smoker's heart because critical blood vessels feeding oxygen to the muscle of his lower heart were clogged with plaque. The procedure is called a Coronary Artery Bypass Graft, or CABG (pronounced "cabbage," like the vegetable). The operation is as intricate and precise, in many ways, as a finely choreographed ballet; surgeons perform more than 300,000 of them every year in the United States, each time cutting deep into the chest, cracking the ribs, and carefully pulling them apart; rerouting the blood to a heart-lung machine that serves as the patient's temporary heart and lungs; replacing diseased vessels with ones still viable; and then closing up the wound.

Scrubbed in with gown, mask, goggles, hood, and cloth covers for my shoes, I watched as a fifth-year resident sliced into Mr. Jacobs's leg to "harvest" a blood vessel. This would later be sewn onto the heart and the coronary artery (which conducts oxygenated blood from the lungs) as a "bypass" around the clogged vessel. The PGY3 was making the final cuts in the chest cavity, carefully removing the pericardial membrane to expose the heart. Both the heart and lungs had stopped functioning, as the patient's medium red blood swirled through a series of clear plastic tubes, perfused with oxygen by a machine with several pistonlike cylinders churning up and down in a chamber filled with blood. One tube conveyed fresh blood to Mr. Jacobs's arterial system; another sucked back out the darker venous blood, depleted of oxygen, returning it to the bypass pump. This allowed the surgeons to operate on the lungs and heart "in stasis," and oddly still.

As the three nurses, two surgical residents, anesthesiologist, two techs, and a perfusionist proceeded in their slow-motion dance, they were pulling down between $15,000 and $50,000 for their hospital—depending on the complexity of the case, how many vessel/bypasses were required, how long the operation took, and what type of insurance the man carried.

The heart surgeon, if he was charging an average fee, billed Mr.

Jacobs in a range from $5,000 to $12,000. The anesthesiologist keeping this fifty-seven-year-old asleep and stable charged between $1,500 and $4,000. The perfusionist, in charge of the heart-lung machine, was paid $90,000 a year, which is more than most*; the senior scrub nurse said she makes $40 an hour; the other nurses said they are paid about $25 an hour. Wages for the orderly who transported the man here, and the women who cleaned up the O.R., range from $6 to $8 an hour.

And what were the residents being paid?

The PGY5, with almost nine years of medical school and residency training behind him, who will be a cardiac fellow next year, earned about $34.00 for this five-hour operation. The PGY3, with almost seven years of intensive postgraduate training and education, realized about $31.25. Both made under $6.80 an hour—$4.30 an hour after taxes—plus benefits.

Obviously, trainees' salary scale should be less than that of a senior physician or technician. One also needs to consider the costs of training and supervising young surgeons in the O.R. Even so, it seems likely the hospital is registering at least a small profit, particularly on the work performed by the PGY5, who in this case was weeks away from finishing his general surgical training and was nearly as qualified as a general surgical attending.

■

It's difficult to muster much sympathy for physicians—even trainees—being underpaid. Not when doctors in the United States fetch an average of $148,000 a year. Yet the fact remains that residents, particularly senior ones, are not paid even close to what they net for hospitals and attendings—or what their equivalent level of education might entitle them to in other professions. From $150 lumbar punctures in the E.R. to $1,500 cardiac catheterizations, from $39 blood drawings to $25,000 heart bypasses, residents are a steal, laboring at $6 to $8 an hour, even after hospital overhead is figured in.

This reminds me of a department chief whose twenty-four-year-old son was finishing business school and about to accept a job at an investment bank. "He will make one-and-a-half times what I pay an assistant professor in the department of medicine," said the chief,

*Other experienced perfusionists I spoke with are paid in the $60,000 range.

sounding amazed. "Now that's right out of two years of business school. My assistant professors have gone through four years of medical school and three years of residency training. We start them in the residency program at $25,000, and they make $26,000 when they leave. They go through three years of fellowship training, and they start at $26,000, and when they leave they make $30,000. They're married. They have one or two children. They start at $50,000 in debt and we pay them an average of $26,000 or $27,000 a year for six years. It's ludicrous."

Admittedly, there is a learning curve involved for residents. But how many $150 lumbar punctures does it take for a $6.50-an-hour intern to get it—three? ten? a thousand? This is especially true for senior residents, who in most hospitals are more expert and efficient than attendings in performing routine, simple bread-and-butter procedures.

None of this would matter if hospitals provided residents with a salary commensurate with their duties, level of education, and competence. In 1993–4, the average salary of a PGY1 was $29,632 plus benefits, a salary that rises about a thousand dollars a year in most programs, this despite the fact that residents are steadily reaping more for their hospital as their proficiency increases. Imagine telling a starting lawyer, banker, or anyone else fresh from professional school that they will be paid five or six dollars an hour for the first three, six, ten, or twelve years of their career. Would they tolerate this? Would the market sustain salaries this low?

This situation is considerably better than forty or fifty years ago, when resident "pay" consisted of only room and board with stipends of a dollar or less a day. Still, it has hardly kept up with the rising cost of living; the fact that residents are no longer predominately young, male, and single; and the dramatic increases in medical school tuition. (In 1986–87, state medical schools' annual tuition averaged $4,574 and private schools $15,023; today these numbers have increased by some 30 percent.) The average debt owed by residents in 1993 was $59,885—more than double the amount a decade earlier—with almost a quarter of all graduates owing more than $75,000. For those whose debt has come due, they may be writing checks for monthly installments equal to more than half the five or six dollars an hour they bring home. Even if they aren't worried about loans coming due, residents training well into their thirties and having families along the way pocket an after-tax income of as little as $200 a week—for up to *nine years.*

Salaries have barely kept up with inflation, with residents earning real, constant dollars at close to the same level they did in 1970. According to an American Association of Medical College study, residents' salaries in 1970 averaged $6,900 a year; in 1992 the number had dropped to $6,100 in constant, 1970 dollars.

"You're making $30,000 and you have a $100,000 debt," said PGY1 Claude Kelly. Kelly, age twenty-seven, has a wife and two small children; and he will not be through until age thirty-four or thirty-five, including a hoped-for subspecialty fellowship. "How are you going to pay that off? I'm scraping the bottom with this debt." He looks agitated to be talking about this, having told me his family of recent Irish immigrants is hardly in a position to help him. "I don't have money for my kids," he says, adding that he frequently agonizes over finances and the prospect of another seven or eight years of meager wages. His wife works but has recently been home with the new baby—and would like to stay there. But she will probably go back to her job, because they need the money. "I'm worried about eating every week," said another married intern at Kelly's hospital. "I'm worried about my old car breaking down, because I can't pay for repairs." One out of three residents moonlight in emergency rooms and clinics—some out of desperation to make ends meet—expanding already onerous schedules to ninety, a hundred, and more hours a week.

The trade-off for exploitation and low wages has long been the promise of a pot of gold at training's end. The fifth-year resident operating on Mr. Jacobs will be worth at least $150,000 as a brand-new general surgeon, almost five times his current compensation as a PGY5. He'll make considerably more if he goes on to complete the fellowship in cardiothoracic surgery he planned to start a few months after this operation. (The average salary for this specialty is over $550,000). Cindy Williams will earn far less as a primary care physician but will still average $80,000 to $100,000 a year, two to three times her current income.

But one has to wonder about the psychological impact of forcing young doctors to endure years of economic hardship. At best, this system encourages physicians to feel entitled to outsized salaries when they finish training, in reward for their long privation—a misguided attitude in this era of cost cutting, when doctors salaries will almost certainly decline, particularly specialists. At worst, it fosters a mentality of "I paid my dues, now they have to pay theirs," a justification residents sometimes hear as attendings seem to vanish at night and on weekends.

■

The simple—and fair—solution would be to align salaries closer to what the market will bear and what residents actually bring in, less what it costs to teach them. But that's the problem. Nobody seems to really know what a residency really costs, which has left the issue open to the usual wide range of philosophies and interpretations.

A few hard-nosed educators think residents should not be paid at all. "I don't see how they can become committed like you have to be if all they're worrying about is making money," a surgical attending and educator in his fifties told me. "You can't be in this for just the money, or you will not be a good doctor." Others believe residents are paid about what they should be. "There is the danger that if we take the salaries up too high," says John Potts of Massachusetts General, "the country will lose its sense of appreciation, that it's truly a training mission." He also believes that too much pay will tarnish a trainee's devotion to medicine. "This is one of the noblest professions there is," he said. "Economics shouldn't be allowed to get in the way of this remarkable dedication. It's old-fashioned, my saying that, but I believe it very strongly. We haven't tried to shove the salary way up because we want to remind people that it's both training and service, and we don't want the service component to get out of balance with the training."

There is also an assumption that residents only *cost* hospitals money—because of their salaries and benefits, added faculty and administrative time, and because they order more tests and may keep patients in the hospital longer. "Residents take time," says William Hazel, the orthopedic surgeon from Virginia. "You can't get as much done. When you put the knife in their hand, you have to watch them. They do help you with rounds, but their economic contribution is not that great."

One study suggests that training residents costs about $50,000 a year per trainee; another says $70,000 a year; still others offer complicated models and formulas to determine costs that can then be passed on to Medicare and other insurers, who currently consider education a legitimate hospital expense. Yet another paper found that patients cared for primarily by residents cost $1,681 per patient more than those cared for by attendings. These patients at Detroit's Henry Ford Medical Center also spent 1.7 more days in the hospital when cared for by trainees. Other studies quantify extra money paid out on tests and procedures, though one conducted in the E.R. of the Medical College of Pennsylvania found that "the presence of a residency training program did not increase the cost of care as measured by test use and, for three of the six diagnoses, actually lowered the cost of care."

Obviously, this data is sketchy and contradictory, yet all these studies, models, and insurance formulas seem to share one basic myth: that the flow of cash is one way, and that residents earn nothing for their institutions.

∎

Over the years, this myth has proven lucrative for teaching hospitals and attendings.* For example, the chief financial officer at Rhode Island Hospital, John Schibler, told me that his hospital received $59 million in 1992 to cover their residency programs— over a quarter of the hospital's $255 million in total revenues. Almost half of this $59 million came from Medicare and Medicaid; the rest was paid as part of patient bills sent to Blue Cross and Blue Shield, HMOs, and other private insurers.

According to Schibler, residents actually cost the hospital $64 million, which he described as a very rough estimate based on accounting models Rhode Island borrowed from other similar-sized hospitals. They used outside data because of the expense and complexity of coming up with their own figures. But even if they had collected their own data, Schibler says they would be only "estimates" based on methodology used by Medicare, including formulas for indirect payments that Schibler admits "nobody really understands.

"If, in fact, we are providing medical education to the tune of $64 million," he said, dividing this amount by the 219 full-time resi-

*Most staff attendings are paid a salary and do not make extra income from patients, either their own or those they attend to with a resident. They do indirectly benefit from residents' taking care of their patients while they do other things. Private attendings, however, can and do charge patients for care rendered by residents.

dents at the hospital, "that works out to, I would say, $290,000 per resident per year."

"That seems really high," I interjected, taken aback by a number about three times what I expected. "Is that what it really costs? Does that include their salary?"

"That would include their salaries," he said, "plus a portion of the faculties' salaries to the extent that they spend time here [with residents]. And there is that additional cost of testing and everything that's involved there; and a portion of the buildings and everything you see around here."

The numbers at Rhode Island are not unique. Nor do I mean to single out this institution as anything but typical. Memos and studies from a half-dozen other academic hospitals verify that this system, and these amounts, exist elsewhere. Indeed, there is a wide range of disbursements that teaching hospitals are paid under the category of resident education. Medicare, for instance, bases its payouts on calculations made in the base year of 1984. According to Tzvi Hefter, director of HCFA's Division of Hospital Services, HCFA figured out what each hospital claimed to be allocating to graduate medical education in 1984, and divided this amount by the number of residents. "Those numbers varied all over the map," said Hefter, "anywhere from $20,000 to $200,000 per resident."

Part of the difference resulted from such factors as numbers of faculty and severity of illness. The rest came from the fact that historically hospitals have assigned their overhead "costs" under a variety of categories. For instance, Rhode Island Hospital in 1984 may have assigned far more of its general costs to its residency program than to its outpatient department, while another hospital did the opposite. This means that when HCFA set out that year to distribute Medicare funds in support of residency programs, some hospitals benefited from the fact they had been assigning more costs to "education" than others.

This is one reason Medicare annually hands over some $90,000 per resident to Rhode Island, while reimbursing some similarly sized programs far less. For instance, Georgetown University Hospital— which has slightly lower revenues, and similar numbers of residents as Rhode Island—receives only about $45,000 per resident.*

---

*I asked an HCFA official if hospitals complained about a system that seems arbitrarily disproportionate. The official said they do complain, but that the law is clear about how the payments are to be decided.

■

In total, Medicare paid some $6.1 billion last year to hospitals for residency programs, a source of income that not only has served as a bulwark to fund graduate medical education in the United States but also has, until recently, encouraged programs to expand house staff positions, in part because each trainee brings in a check from the government. In 1993, an article in the *Journal of the American Osteopathic Association* titled "A Primer on Graduate Medical Education Financing," advised education program directors to "Sign on as many residents as possible," claiming that disbursements from the government were so generous that a program could expect to turn a profit. "Current regulations and payment mechanisms support funding and filling as many resident spots as the institution can adequately train," explains the article. "Total reimbursement for each added resident generally exceeds any extra incremental costs to the hospital."

Another article in the *Journal of General Internal Medicine* reports that doubling the number of residents and fellows at the Western Pennsylvania Hospital in Pittsburgh, from eighteen to thirty-six trainees, resulted in reimbursements that not only offset the additional costs of resident salaries, hiring new faculty, and so forth, but also produced a net *profit*. "We conclude," write the authors, "that expanding the medical residency resulted in additional net revenue to the hospital in excess of the increase in measured costs."

In fact, this was exactly what was supposed to happen, according to Tzvi Hefter. He said the idea of handing out a set amount of money each year is to stimulate efficiency by encouraging programs to spend less than what they are paid, so they can pocket the difference. "This is the name of the game," he said, adding that Medicare has long encouraged the expansion of residency programs, since until recently it was considered in the public's interest to train more doctors. "This policy," he said, "is being reviewed right now in Congress," which almost certainly will be cutting this stipend for teaching hospitals—and may have already done so when this book is published.

When I told one of the residency directors at Rhode Island that the hospital says it got paid upwards of $290,000 per resident, he said, "No way. If that's true, I want to know where that money goes, because it sure doesn't come to me." A surgical resident responded, "That's gotta be hogwash." He had just finished sewing up a laceration in the E.R. for which the hospital would bill, he guessed, $250 to $300—while paying him $2.50 or so for twenty minutes of his time.

■

We can't let all of this eye-glazing talk of studies and arbitrary formulas obscure a central truth—that the success of teaching hospitals as paragons of the "triple terror" is possible because residents have long performed the lion's share of patient care on the wards. "The profit that doctors and hospitals derived from house staff was one of the driving forces of the postwar medical system," writes sociologist Paul Starr, in his Pulitzer Prize–winning book, *The Social Transformation of American Medicine.* Indeed, Starr reports that a prominent hospital in New England once tried to "tax" private attendings who used residents to tend to their hospitalized patients free of charge. "Since the house staff performed services for which the practitioners often charged fees, this idea might not seem unreasonable," intimates Starr. "Of course, the ensuing uproar among the private physicians caused the proposal to be withdrawn."

Not surprisingly, given this point of view, Starr argues that it is the financial attractiveness of residents as much as a commitment to education that has led to sizable gaps between the supply and demand of trainees. Every year, hospitals fail to fill 30 to 40 percent of their residency slots—even with thousands of foreign medical graduates specially imported to swell the rolls. Last year, America's teaching hospitals wanted 20,751 first-year residents but got only about 13,000 graduating from American medical schools, and about 3,000 from abroad—a gap that will almost certainly grow worse, given widespread calls for medical schools to cut back on enrollees in an age of doctor surplus. Congress is also calling for reductions in visas issued to foreign medical graduates to work as residents.

Perhaps this disparity in supply and demand indicates a resident's true financial worth to a hospital faced with hiring either a $30,000-a-year resident who toils three times harder than anyone else, or another $100,000 attending, or a $40,000 nurse or technician. Another possible indicator of a resident's true value (and earning power) is moonlighting. Typically, community hospitals who lack residents but need to maintain E.R.'s and clinics around the clock pay $50 to as much as $100 an hour for licensed residents and fellows. These fees acknowledge services rendered, and are calculated not by hospitals setting arbitrary "stipends" but by what the market will bear.

Medical educators are taking some measures to alleviate the inequities of service versus education. Recently, the Accreditation Council for Graduate Medical Education, the main body overseeing and accrediting residency programs, has cracked down on a few of the worse exploiters. Last year, they put dozens of residency programs on probation, or withdrew or withheld accreditation. One of the major reasons, according to John Gienapp, executive director of the ACGME, stems from letting education in these programs be subsumed by service and scut. Last year, for instance, the ACGME stripped accreditation from orthopedic surgery programs in two New York City hospitals—Lincoln Medical and Mental Health Center in the South Bronx, and Metropolitan Hospital Center in East Harlem—because residents were being overworked and received little or no education in these busy inner-city facilities. "This doesn't happen very often," said Steven Nestler, secretary of the residency review committee for orthopedic surgery at the ACGME. "The residents are supposed to be learning. But they can't be so busy taking care of patients that no one is teaching them anything. That may be what's going on here."

Last year, the ACGME announced it will be tightening up its review process and enforcement of rules, including specific requirements that education take precedence over service. It's unclear what this means for residents enduring long hours of scut, service, and minimum-wage labor, though Gienapp claims that "moving residencies more in the direction of education" is increasingly a high priority.

He admits this will not be easy. "American residents are still more service driven than, let's say, in Canada," says Gienapp, adding that "financially we cannot get the top decision makers to hire $30,000 phlebotomists* when you have residents doing this work already, and their costs are reimbursed by the government."

∎

---

*Technicians trained to draw blood and place I.V.'s.

Meanwhile, after sixteen minutes of looking for her X ray, Cindy Williams launched phase two of her quest: finding someone to read the film. Blasting down the hall from the rays record room, with her long coat again trailing like a billowing cloud, Williams went searching for a radiologist. Without breaking stride, she turned back to me and flashed a lethal look. "Keep that timer going," she said. "This scut run's not through yet."

CHAPTER 7

For the Love of Medicine

All my life, I wanted to be a doctor. Now I'm tired. I'm burned out. I'm just not so sure. Maybe I should have been a lawyer.

Third-year resident

I t's a common suspicion that doctors go into medicine because they want to get rich, or because they love to be in control—or both. But the truth is that many aspiring physicians launch their training filled with idealism, only to lose it by the time they finish.

"*I'm* not going to get cynical," insists Carol Tisch, a brand new M.D., just three weeks out from earning her medical degree. Tough and exuberant at 1:30 A.M., Carol told me she was on call in her hospital's orthopedic ward not to make big money someday, but because of a passion for surgery. At twenty-eight, she speaks mostly in short, clipped sentences, as if talking were a waste of time when she could be *doing* something—like operating. On her very first rotation as a resident, Carol stands with feet spread and shoulders erect; a short woman with the posture of a defensive lineman poised to absorb any blow, and give one back, if necessary.

Twenty hours after stepping onto the ward near dawn this morning, Carol admits she's weary, telling me that she has been too excited and busy to sleep much during the first few days of her residency. Still, she manages an impressive enthusiasm, given the time of night. She bounds up and down the halls checking charts, double- and triple-checking that labs were taken and drugs administered, and carrying around a four-inch-thick textbook of orthopedic surgery she plans to read this week. "I won't sleep tonight," she says, tying up her thin black hair into a ponytail like a man might roll up his sleeves before going to work. "But it's early in the course of things. Later on, I probably won't be able to do this." The only dark edge to her new life, she says, is her fiancé. A neurologist she

149

met in medical school, he is four years her senior, and already finished with his training. "He gripes about not having the things that
a traditional husband would have, I guess," she says, noting she
wishes she had that kind of support, too. "He calls me up and tor-
tures me on the phone when I'm on call. But I can't be there as
much as I have been in medical school." They had no immediate
plans to marry, or to have children.

By morning, Carol is still remarkably vibrant, standing in the fil-
tered, slightly cooled air of an operating room. Wrapped like everyone else in green scrubs, gloves, thick gown, mask, and face shield,
she is closing up an incision cut into a sixty-six-year-old former
automobile assembly line worker with arthritis in his left hip so
severe he could no longer walk. The attending, Charles Reynolds,
has just inserted a new hip, and finished sewing up the muscles and
tendons severed as part of the operation. Knowing Carol is a tenderfoot, he watches as she carefully punctures the skin around the
wound with a long, half-circle-shaped needle, pulling the incision
closed with a thin blue thread. She's slow and shaking ever so
slightly, but she gains confidence with each new stitch. Halfway
through, Reynolds turns away to answer a page, apparently confident she can work a moment or two without him.

Afterward, Carol is giddy. "Reynolds is known for being tough as
nails," she said. "Did you see that? He didn't say a thing. No
insults. No telling me I was screwing it up."

As I left her later that afternoon, I remember thinking, "If anyone
is going to make it, Carol Tisch will."

■

I didn't see Dr. Tisch again for over a year, catching up with her
during the fall of her second year. I had been keeping up with her
now and then by phone, and knew her zeal had diminished somewhat as fatigue and the grind of internship took its toll. But I was
not prepared—I never am—to see her afflicted with what has
become a sadly familiar ashen complexion and tired eyes, clearly
visible despite a layer of makeup (she had worn little or none before
that I could remember). She was just coming off a 36-hour shift—
and two months of what she claimed were 130-hour weeks at an
outerlying hospital affiliated with her program.

"Things haven't gone exactly as I envisioned," she mentioned over coffee and stale cake in the hospital's cafeteria. "You get beat down. You're like a fetus growing but instead of maturing, you mutate. In ways you didn't expect. And don't like." I asked what happened, and she leaned in close to whisper. "It's lots of things. Mostly the attitudes. I hold pretty high standards for myself, but I can see that this is the type of thinking that has led to the behavior patterns in a lot of my attendings. Perfection. Demanding. Unforgiving. I'm trying to avoid these characteristics in myself. It does have to be grueling to a point because some of it can really stun you, what can go wrong.

"I'm very competitive, so it's an endurance race," she added. "Everybody tries to do a better job than everybody else for a longer period of time. We all feel for our patients—most of us, anyway— but the fact is when you reach a certain level of fatigue, the thing that keeps you going is *not* your concern for the patient. I hate to admit it. It's the knowledge that someone senior to you who has expectations of you, and, by God, you better not fail them." This means mostly being in the O.R., she said, and leaving patients hanging on the floors with only an intern present. "But it's the patients on the floor who are suffering, and this bothers me. You can excel in one area, but you're failing in another."

She cited several examples, including one day when she was the sole doctor assigned to the Surgical Intensive Care Unit (SICU) who was not in the O.R. On the floor she was having trouble with an elderly patient post-op from abdominal surgery, when the woman suddenly stopped breathing. She needed to be intubated fast. "I knew I was in way over my head on this one," said Carol, explaining that she tried to "scratch the throat"—cut it with a scalpel to insert the breathing tube—but it didn't work. "So you take the tube out, do it again. Same thing. Check everything. Everything's okay, and again the patient deteriorates. And it turns out it's just a little finesse move [she was unaware of] with the stylette, which is a little instrument that you use to guide in your tube." Tisch says she eventually called in help, and that the patient survived. But this shouldn't have happened, she said, adding that the incident shook up her confidence for a while—in part because she felt unprepared.

She talked about the rotation she had just finished at the other hospital. "I went out there," she says, "and suddenly six critically ill patients are foisted on me, and I'm to oversee two brand-new, green interns out on the floor, and I have a senior who is a mad dog. He wants to keep people alive who could be growing mold. Do you have any idea how much time and money and effort that consumes, keeping a body alive that wants to die?" Carol said this senior resident, a PGY4, had just finished two years in a lab, working on a research project. "Understandably, he wanted to operate all day. He wanted to make a big splash. This is his personality I'm talking about. Death cannot be allowed to win. It was inhumane. So he had us working 140, 150 hours a week for 8 weeks." I asked if she ever complained.

"You can voice it, but you still do what you're told. You can't refuse. I hate to admit it, but if you have very strong moral, ethical groundings, you're probably not in surgery. It's like being in the military. It's very much a hierarchical system. The chairman [of the department] is your general. But in each section you've got the potential for your own little Hitler." Indeed, Carol Tisch says she follows orders because more than anything she wants to be a surgeon—a craving so powerful it sometimes scares her. "I'm telling you, it's an affliction," she intimates, vowing that when she finishes, she will be more humane. "I'm not going to be like that," she whispers hopefully, though clearly Carol Tisch is worried she will be swept into the very attitudes she finds so troubling.

I asked if being a woman made a difference, knowing that a couple of my female friends who had gone into surgery were having serious second thoughts. "It's very tough for a woman in surgery," she said. "We have far fewer than in medicine, and it's still old boy to the max. Macho. It's stupid, but that's the way it is."

In general medicine, I told Carol, some educators have told me they think women have been a great influence, making this specialty more humane and their residency less macho. She laughed. "That's what I hear. But in surgery, forget it. Hasn't happened."

This reminded me of a friend in the Midwest, another highly competitive woman who took two years off from a surgical residency to conduct research and to spend more time with her husband and new baby. She was terrified to go back and miss the time with her family. Another woman friend in the Southwest quit surgery altogether, switching after a year of soul-searching to anesthesiology. Hiking one day in the mountains, she told me she still wanted to be a surgeon, but that the price was too high.

I asked Carol how things were going with her fiancé, and she grimaced. "He's history," she said. "Couldn't cope. Now, it's just me and my dog. You have to be very much your own best company and your own best support, because people around you don't understand what's going on. Literally, you lose control. You've got these creditors knocking at your door because you don't have the energy to open your mail. It's unbelievable the way things fall apart."

Finishing her snack, Carol told me it was her birthday. "I'm thirty-one," she said, suddenly sounding very sad, almost as if she would cry. She maintained her composure, though, and told me she was going home to celebrate with her collie. "*He* doesn't even know me anymore," she said, smiling wanly with lips dolloped in lipstick.

■

Educators who pay attention to these things have long lamented what one called "the loss of innocence" during a physician's training. Robert Ebert, former dean of Harvard Medical School, talks about "those stalwart physicians who persevere" through their training but "often lose their idealism." Steve Bergman—a.k.a. Samuel Shem, author of *The House of God,* who went on after his internship at Beth Israel Hospital in Boston to become a psychiatrist and professor at Harvard Medical School—talks about the first two years of medical school. "These kids are so full of optimism and compassion," he says. "Then the third year comes, and they go to these big institutions all around town and they start to really get crushed. I've seen it for years now, how they get brutalized." He tells about a student who was rounding with his medical team one morning and noticed a patient's bed was empty, a woman he had helped care for a day earlier. "When he asked what happened," says Bergman, "they said, 'Oh, she died.' Boom. And it's a little thing, and there are a lot worse examples. The point is by the middle of that year, these students who were open and eager and idealistic, they are closing down, and getting cynical, suspicious, tight, already kind of burned out. I can almost tell a fourth-year student from a beginning third-year just by looking at him. I can tell from the body language."

Part of this has to do with the shock and intensity of a young, healthy person's being confronted by illness and disease for the first time—AIDS victims, drug addicts, kids with terminal cancer. "As a resident, you are not only learning how to be a doctor," said Ed Iannuccilli, who recently retired as director of medical education at Rhode Island Hospital. "You're also learning how to be an adult. You are learning how to prioritize, not only in treating and managing patients but in handling yourself. Learning to turn on and off the intensity. How to relax. How to take care of yourself and to realize you're mortal."

"But the system makes this very, very hard," says Bergman, "by working you far harder than you need to learn medicine, and by ignoring compassion too often. You come away with scars."

■

This does not have to happen. Indeed, it can be countered to some extent by the satisfaction that only a physician can know—of bringing to bear skills, intelligence, grit, and art to help someone truly and profoundly. There is also the intense sense of accomplishment when a surgeon makes the right cut, or the medicine intern the right diagnosis, and suddenly an ill or dying baby, or grandfather, or somebody's little sister recovers—their wan face turning pink again, their eyes turning from glazed to lucent.

Take Rich Ferrara, the anesthesiology fellow who watched in horror as a surgical fellow accidentally punctured a forty-seven-year-old woman's pulmonary artery. This episode and others naturally left him feeling cynical and sad about what can happen when the system breaks down, in this case compounded when surgeons apparently covered up a fatal lapse in judgment by not telling the family, and convincing them to bury their mother without an autopsy.

"I don't want you to get the impression that there is no satisfaction in medicine," Ferrara says evenly. "What makes it all okay is the patients, knowing you did something to help. You try to focus on this, and not the bad things."

He remembered back to his sixth week of internship, when he was a brand-new M.D. He had a patient in her sixties, near death from a cancerous tumor that was literally eating away her bones. The surgeons wanted to try one more operation, but there was a problem. "She was a very frail lady who looked like she would just crumble if you touched her. She had white hair, blotchy skin. I think she had multiple myeloma. She basically had mush for bones."

Even though this woman had only six weeks to live, a surgeon decided she needed a bilateral total hip replacement, where both hips are entirely removed and replaced by prosthetic hips. "She hadn't been out of bed for three months because she had such hip pain, and she went to see an orthopedic surgeon and he said, 'Let's do your hips. You'll be able to walk again.' This was one of those guys who would basically operate on a dead person, for the money and experience of it."

Ferrara did not agree with the operation, and tried to dissuade the patient. Because the woman's bones were so weak, Ferrara and his attending were worried about putting a breathing tube down her throat while she was fully sedated, since it involved tipping back a neck that might snap without the alert patient's muscle tension to hold it in place.

"I told this lady in very stark terms the risks, but she was just adamant. The surgeon had promised her she would walk again, and she really wanted to walk. So I said, 'Okay, if this is what you really, really want, I'll do everything in my power to make it go safely.' So I spent that entire weekend practicing so I could do the most painless, accurate laryngoscopy on an awake patient. Putting the blade in the mouth and lifting it up so I could put the tube in. I took a dummy home with me, and worked until I had the procedure down to about a minute and a half. I was so terrified of doing this and making her uncomfortable. It really meant a lot to me because this was such a foolish operation, and I was determined to be her advocate and protect her because that's what she wanted.

"I had learned to intubate patients under controlled circumstances," he said. "Asleep patients with good airways, with an attending standing over me. This was going to be awake. I felt like I had no business doing this, but my attending that day said I was ready and insisted on me doing everything that day, and he watched but would not get into it.

"I was incredibly nervous," he said when they wheeled the old woman into the O.R., so fragile in a pink hospital gown. She was mildly sedated with 1 mg of midazolam, a Valium-like drug, and half a mg of droperidol, which dries up certain bodily secretions to keep the breathing tube clear.

"I was standing behind her," says Ferrara, "so she's lying down on her back, and her head is elevated just a little bit on some pillows and I'm standing behind her forehead, looking down. I say, 'okay, Mrs.—

I won't use her name—I'm opening up your mouth now and I want you to stick out your tongue, now I'm putting the blade back here and this is going to be uncomfortable.' And I sprayed up her mouth with a little bit of lidocaine and then I said: 'I'm going to lift up your tongue and now I'm seeing the back of your throat, and now I'm seeing your tonsils, and now I'm seeing your arytenoids, and there are the vocal cords and, okay now, Mrs. Whatever, you are going to feel a little squirt,' and I gave her more lidocaine, and I slid that tube right down there, 'you are going to feel us helping you breathe, and now I want you to help us turn you over.' "

Ferrara says the woman watched him the entire time, her eyes wide with anxiety and concentration.

"I was so junior," he remembered. "It was like jumping off the lip of a mountain and hoping the snow is going to meet your skis and that you're going to be able to keep going." The entire operation was very intense, he says. "The whole thing went about twelve hours, but I wouldn't even leave the room. I wouldn't take a lunch break or anything like that because I was determined to stand by this lady."

The operation was a success, as they say, though the patient died—some two weeks later, from her cancer. The woman did not get her wish of walking again, but she was able to sit up in bed, something her son told Ferrara meant a lot to her.

" 'She appreciated all the care that you took and the concern for her dignity, and her safety,' " Ferrara says the son told him. " 'She appreciated how much you were willing to follow her wishes even though that wasn't what you thought was the best alternative for her.' "

Ferrara says he will never forget the gratitude in the dying woman's eyes, and in those of her son. "I was really moved by the whole thing, because it taught me about patients and their need for dignity, and because I was able to use what little I knew to make it go as well as possible for her.

" 'She was terrified about you putting that tube in her awake,' " the son said to Ferrara, " 'because you had described it in such vivid detail to her, but she had so much trust in you that there was no way she was going to let anyone else do that but you.' "

As he left the son after this last meeting, Rich Ferrara's eyes teared up. "I felt like this validated everything I am trying to do. It makes up for all the bad things. It's a high like nothing else."

■

Personal epiphanies, says philosopher Stephen Vicchio, are rare in medicine, but less rare than for most people. Even so, if surveys are any indication, Rich Ferrara's "high like nothing else" does not happen often enough to offset deep disappointments many physicians say they feel after residency—deflations that begin during training, and for many continue beyond.

Experts who counsel physicians and monitor their attitudes toward themselves and their profession insist that doctors are feeling burned out, angry, and even depressed in unprecedented numbers. "I know there is a lot of pain out there," says John-Henry Pfifferling, director of the Center for Professional Well-Being in Durham, North Carolina, and a nationally known speaker and consultant to physician groups and hospitals. "There are a lot of docs who are facing burnout, who are having trouble holding on to the passion that brought them to medicine."

In a poll of young physicians taken by the AMA, doctors under age forty, or who had been in practice seven years or less, were asked: "Given what you know about medicine as a career, if you were in college today, would you go to medical school?" An astonishing one out of three said no; another one out of ten said they weren't sure. Another study reports that almost 51 percent of physicians would not recommend medicine as a career for their own children. Other surveys and polls claim that 91 percent of young physicians say their family life has suffered from the emotional demands of their jobs; 70 percent of doctors feel pessimistic that the future of health care will not improve their roles as physicians; and on and on.

"I've seen this number before," said surgeon William Hazel, talking about the 40 percent of young physicians who are unhappy with their choice of medicine as a career. "I think it's accurate." Hazel also served as chairperson of the young physicians section of the AMA in 1991–92.

He attributed this negativity in large part to the way physicians are trained, both the deprivations and the lack of preparation for what they will face when they leave the rarefied world of a large teaching hospital and enter the real world of medicine. "You go in with a set of expectations," he says, "and then the game changes. If you expected to go out and make a lot of money and have autonomy, or if you just expected to see patients and go home, you're disillusioned." He said that his residency, like most, virtually ignored economics, management training, and other skills he says are critical to understanding the practical side of medicine—and how to cope with the tremendous structural changes happening in health care.

Hazel was even more concerned with the value system he was exposed to during his residency, however. "We are taught how to be great doctors technically. But there's more to it. There is the emotional realm and there's the spiritual realm, and I think maybe we've lost some of that somewhere. I'm almost an addict for working hard, because that's what we're taught to do. But when I see that it's easier for a patient to reach me than for my wife and kids, I feel like I've gotten away from balancing things that are important."

When he completed medical school and residency, Hazel said, "It was like I had been away for nine years, and then suddenly I was finished, and there was my wife and our kids, nine years older. I felt like this time had been taken from me, and I wanted to change this, but I'm finding it hard. I love medicine, but I also love life. The two should not be incompatible."

"I think doctors are socialized early on to be arrogant," said Tom Delbanco, chief of medicine and primary care at Beth Israel Hospital in Boston. Of British origin, the soft-spoken, bearded Delbanco has spent several years studying the attitudes and beliefs of doctors and patients. "They are brought up from day one to feel privileged and special, if not by the public anymore, then by their peers. Their peers both denigrate them and clobber them in their training, but at the same time tell them how special and wonderful they are, the teachers. And it takes a lot to get them off that pedestal, and they don't like falling off it. It's a rude awakening, and they're getting very rude awakenings these days."

■

This was particularly poignant for Mark Stafford, an internist formerly in a family practice in Dothan, Alabama. Twelve years ago, as he emerged from his residency at the University of Alabama, he entered private practice in this rural town famous for its peanuts, convinced that if he plunged heart and soul into his patients' care, they would venerate and admire him. "I threw everything into my work," Stafford says, "and ended up caring too much and giving more to my patients than I could expect them to give me in return." Gradually, he says, this wore him down, coming to a head one afternoon when he was summoned to his local hospital to cover the patients of a close friend, a cardiologist killed that day in a motorcycle accident.

By the time he arrived on the wards that day, recalls Stafford, "all these patients knew their doctor had died. Yet I was struck by them saying in one breath, 'I'm really sorry to hear about our doctor,' and in the next asking, 'but what are you going to do about my laxative?' 'What are you going to do about my medication?' And I thought, Here's a person who gave everything he had, and at his death, all people could think about were their own needs." Crushed by this experience, Stafford gave up on private practice and returned to Alabama's medical school in Birmingham, where he now tells students and residents that they must learn that "patients aren't always there to support you. You are performing a service, nothing more and nothing less."

William Porter, a fifty-seven-year-old oncologist and professor of medicine at Carolinas Medical Center in Charlotte, North Carolina, also gave up private practice and returned to an academic setting, burned out by the intensity of coping with severely ill cancer patients. "It exacts at least a pound and a half of flesh for every encounter to do it right," he says, "to be a resource to sick and dying patients, to be compassionate." Porter adds that initially he went into cancer treatment because, during residency, he was fascinated by the science of dealing with it, which was "all that mattered in an academic setting. I was so in love with just the science of medicine that I thought I could sort of drag along the humanism. But it didn't work out that way."

At first, Porter embraced the challenge of caring for the very sick. But after a while, it overwhelmed him. "You are seeing patients whose prognosis you recognize is so bad that the kindest thing would be to offer them only comfort care. But that is a profoundly unacceptable formulation for most people, so you find yourself enrolling them in clinical trials that are barbaric or offering them chemotherapy as almost a placebo. You do this enough times, and it can harden your heart, until it becomes theater rather than human-to-human interaction. You become an actor in your own play, and you can loathe yourself for the kind of insincerity that is at the heart of your own enterprise. It might be quite successful theater, but it doesn't really proceed out of a kind of shared humaneness and a shared compassion, because you've got this dirty little secret that you've tried to share with them and they're not willing to hear."

Porter adds that many doctors, including himself, expect—even yearn for—a certain lifestyle and income, only to discover that the work is less fulfilling than they anticipated. Few have the where-withal to escape, however, as Porter did, accepting a huge cut in salary to return to the cloister, in a sense. "It's really ironic," he says. "I'm over here preparing young doctors for the kind of life I left, when I know damn well they're heading into the jaws of a health care system which will chew 'em up and spit 'em out within a very short time unless something's found to change the quality of what they do. But I don't tell them that. I don't paint that pessimistic a picture. I try to warn them about taking care of themselves, and not to be so obsessed with money and with the volume that they get over-whelmed, making sure they keep their stamp collection going, or their lovers, or whatever it takes to get them through the night."

Most physicians I have met are not this gloomy. Some even seemed to welcome the intense environment Porter fled from, thriving on tending the very ill—delighted to forgo the old imperative of making money, and living high on the pedestal of self-perceived power and prestige. Tom Delbanco talks about AIDS, saying that in the absence of any significant medical cure, "The most important thing you can do is care, like old-fashioned healers, which can be very fulfilling for a certain type of doctor."

There are plenty of physicians who have found great fulfillment in working quietly in a small town in family practice, or working overseas in refugee camps, or even working on staff for HMOs—who are taught, or innately know, or manage to retain despite everything a sense of balance between humility and firmness, com-passion and fortitude. However, if the experts and polls are to be believed, these well-balanced doctors are in the minority today.

■

Lately, some educators have begun to recognize that the double bane of privation and the pedestal is outmoded and dangerously out of step with medicine's current reality. For instance, not long ago Tom Delbanco and several colleagues launched a series at Boston's Beth Israel they've dubbed "clinical crossroads," which each month investigates a patient's case, presenting not only the science of their disease but also "the psychosocial, economic, and environmental circumstances of the patient, information about the doctor caring for the patient," and the "crossroads" faced by the doctor and patient in treating the whole of their situation.

In 1995, Delbanco, et. al. began publishing their cases in *The Journal of the American Medical Association*—an approach that updates an idea launched in 1906 when a Harvard physician named Richard Cabot initiated a series of "whodunit" case studies in Boston. These evolved into the famous "Case Records of the Massachusetts General Hospital," published once a week in *The New England Journal of Medicine*. In an age when being a physician means far more than knowing a patient's BUN, or diagnosing his renal disease, Delbanco's case studies should serve as a model for educators who want their young charges to avoid the malaise felt by some of their seniors.

Another positive development is the nascent movement in residency programs to increase the time trainees spend in clinics and ambulatory care settings, where patients are not all hooked up to machines, and the problems both medical and psychosocial are closer to what residents will experience after they finish their training. Despite these innovations, however, the overwhelming emphasis remains on heavy-duty hospital care, with residents living and learning—and sometimes being exploited and abused—in the same claustral world of fatigue and intensity that ill served William Hazel, Mark Stafford, and William Porter.

■

I was thinking about Hazel and the others late in 1994, when I visited a regional meeting of the American Medical Students Association (AMSA) at Tufts University School of Medicine in Boston. These students represented not only the future of medicine, but a new and unexpected development: the sudden revival of interest among young people in being a physician. Indeed, for almost a decade and a half, between 1975 and 1989, interest as measured in applications to medical schools had been in a steep decline, bottoming out in 1988, when only 26,721 people applied for 17,108 positions—down from 42,000 in 1974.

In 1994, however, 46,000 applied—an all-time record—despite the uncertainties in medicine today and the widespread frustration of those in practice. Obviously, this trend reflects even greater uncertainties in recently attractive fields such as business and law, yet at least one member of this new class of doctor candidates has speculated that he and his fellow students are motivated by idealism and a desire "for an experience that seems increasingly hard to come by." Writing in the *New York Times,* Harvard medical student David Shaywitz tried to explain his generation's motivations. "Being a doctor is not as glamorous as it seems on TV shows like *E.R.,*" he wrote, "but it is very personal, immediate and real. You don't spend your days trying to persuade people to buy a product or a service. Your interaction is of a completely different nature."

Young, bright, and practically bouncing in their chairs with ebullience, the AMSA students I spoke with wholeheartedly represented this sentiment. Sitting around a circular table in Tufts's cafeteria, they talked about helping people, about why it was wrong to go into medicine to earn lots of money, and about how they constituted "a new breed" of healers because their medical schools, Tufts University and the University of Pittsburgh, were stressing ethics and patient interaction skills. They were also proud of the fact that their schools were enrolling more women and minorities. "There's an emphasis on human touch and patient interaction, said twenty-four-year-old Jason Emmick, a second-year medical student at Pittsburgh. "It may be an egotistical way of looking at it, but it feels like we are in the front wave of breaking down these barriers."

"I love the idea of taking something that is on the edge of technology," added Gus Emmick, Jason's twenty-three-year-old brother, a second-year at Tufts, "and being able to provide it to an individual person, hopefully making their life better. That's why I'm going into medicine."

I asked if anyone in the group was in medicine to get rich. They seemed surprised by the question, insisting that it was too much work and stress to go through just for money. "You can pay me all the money in the world," said Shanna Miskovsky, twenty-three, another second-year at Pittsburgh, "but if I didn't like what I was doing, forget it."

The oldest of the group was a single mother at Tufts, a second-year named Yvonne Imani. She had been a nurse, and knew more than the others about the reality of life in a hospital. "I've ventured out there before," she said quietly, after listening to the others talk. "I know what it's like. I've been put to tears before. It happens. I've heard from third-year students that there is a resident around here that brags about being the worst there is, it's like a tradition. And so you have people who are monsters and people out there who are nice." She turned to Jason and added: "I was going to say what you said, that we are the beginning of the front wave, but it's going to take time before it kicks in. There's going to be class after class before it kicks in."

I asked if they were worried about their third-year clerkships—if the hours and the "monsters" would alter them, or dampen their optimism.

Yvonne said she's going to fight it. "I'm going to keep my empathy. You have to have empathy. You can't lose that one."

"Maybe that's the difference between being a doctor and a healer," said twenty-six-year-old Laura Smith, a first-year at Pittsburgh. "There has to be a difference," she added, "doesn't there?"

■

Not all residents buy into the idea that empathy, touch, and bedside manner are as important as, say, knowing precisely where to cut when repairing an inguinal hernia, or how to cauterize a blood vessel properly. "I cannot conceive of this sort of kinder, gentler version of surgery," claimed Randy Gaines, a fourth-year surgical resident at one of the more traditional programs in the United States. The son of a surgeon, Gaines was short and blond, displaying wire-rim glasses and a tendency to deliver sermons on why a surgical residency must be akin to running a gauntlet of arrows and fire. Jim Hargrove, a PGY2 I was tailing at the time, described him as "a surgeon who talks too much for a surgeon."

"I think anything that tries to make the training less rigorous would be bad for surgery," said Gaines, weighing the Bell Regulations and other reforms that would lessen hours and change the residency as practiced in his conservative program. "Basically, you need to know your stuff. And I really think that when someone needs a surgeon, they aren't concerned about how empathetic they are. The surgeon may be a son-of-a-bitch, but if he's good, that's who you're going to want cutting into you."

To Gaines, part of the experience includes routinely razzing interns, and generally behaving as if he was far more macho than thou. As I followed his team for morning rounds, he frequently chewed out the PGY1 on call, who had been up and frantic on the surgical ward all night. "Don't make that mistake again," Gaines snapped when the PGY1 was slow in responding to a question. When he hesitated once more, Gaines turned to me and said in a loud voice: "You hear that whistle in the air? That's a cruise missile. It just flew over this intern's bow. The next one is gonna hit, dead on." A few minutes later, Gaines and another senior resident were after the PGY1 again, telling him that in the old days, "when giants walked these halls, they would have impaled you on a sword for saying such a thing."

Other than the intern, everyone on the team smiled and treated Gaines's comments as jokes. In fact, there seemed to be the sort of intense camaraderie and bonding among those on the team that one sees in the military—which Gaines told me later was part of the reason for what he called "the banter." But the intern—the new guy, who was clearly frazzled—did not smile. He looked miserable.

I asked Gaines why he was doing this. He said it was part of the drill, necessary to hammer home the idea of responsibility. "You are captain of the ship, and we kind of joke about it in cardiac surgery that if you make the wrong decision, then the patient's heart gets broken. But there are a lot of times when that's actually true. If Dr. R. [the intern] gets the heart opened up and starts putting stitches in it and he can't get it closed, the heart starts to fall apart, and that's it."

I pointed out that Dr. R. wasn't operating on anybody's heart at the moment, and was only guilty of being a little sluggish. "Excuses are monuments to nothing. The point of it is not to razz them," said Gaines. "The point is to teach them how to be surgeons. I think as the intern I have to have a militaristic view. For instance, I had one of the interns tell me yesterday, 'On Mrs. So-and-so, you wanted me to get another blood culture.' She said, 'I couldn't get one. She doesn't have any veins.' I said to her, 'That's not an acceptable answer. You have to learn a surgeon doesn't do that.' "

As I followed Gaines about that day, he insisted his hard-line approach would benefit his patients, ensuring that they got the best care possible. "What we are teaching is not discipline for discipline's sake. The biggest thing you've got to learn is the surgeon's responsibility to his patient. A lot of that's being accountable for every detail. Knowing every lab, having checked it, having looked at it. Why? Because you're responsible for it. You get the job done."

Gaines's philosophy of total immersion meant he spent virtually every waking moment in the hospital, despite having a wife and baby boy whom he says he doesn't get to see very much. "I think you have to marry someone who's particularly understanding and self-sacrificing," he said, "who understands this is what you have to do. She better be bright enough to know this, to know that if it's a Saturday, and I'm off, and I hear there's a triple A on our service, I'll be right in." He said this was especially true if it was his patient. "Ain't nobody going to cover for me." Gaines said he was home so little he didn't even know where his wife shopped or banked. "I don't know how much money I'm making," he said. "My wife handles all that, because I need to be here."

That night, there were no surgeries planned for Gaines's service, but he stayed late anyway, eating pizza with the other guys and watching a basketball game in the surgeon's lounge. I pointed out to him and the others that they might be home right now, with their families. "Why are you here?" I asked.

There was a moment of silence. "I don't have a good answer for that," said the PGY2, Jim Hargrove, who is married. Gaines, though, did. He said he was there so he wouldn't miss anything. "What if a big case comes through the door?"

This made me wonder if part of Gaines's motivation was simply the thrill of being here—of belonging to what is essentially one of the most exclusive clubs in the world, to be genuinely learning a craft, even as he was slowly being initiated into a culture as rarefied as any medieval aristocracy or royal clique.

Maybe this *is* all necessary. Maybe Gaines is right, and surgeons and to some extent all physicians must go through this initiation to become tough enough to handle what they need to, and to be obsessed with being there all the time—whether it's for one's patients, or simply for the thrill of it all. Yet I wonder what will happen when Gaines crosses the finish line, as William Hazel and

Mark Stafford have done. These doctors had come out as excellent technicians but found themselves lacking in other critical areas their training had ignored. (This would include finances, which Gaines can afford to ignore while he's training, letting his wife bank for him, but he will need to know something about it once he is out.) What would happen once the prop of the team and the training culture was gone, and Gaines and his fellow residents had to stand on their own?

■

In 1993, Bill Moyers spoke at length with Tom Delbanco on the PBS special *Healing and the Mind*. Moyers, after watching Delbanco work with patients, said: "I get the sense that you treat the body and appeal to the mind. Is that a fair characterization?"

"I hope I'm addressing both the body and the mind," said Delbanco. "But they're so intertwined that it's hard for me to differentiate. I know more about the body than the mind. It's probably easier to study, and that's why we learned it in medical school—ninety-five percent body and five percent mind. But I'll tell you, once you're in practice, and you're taking care of real people, it becomes much closer to fifty-fifty."

Delbanco contends that physicians must be taught to understand their patients beyond the body, that the "fun of being a doctor is being trained in the science of medicine and the art of medicine, and then bringing those elements together with the mystery of being a healer."

"But how do you bring mystery and art together with science?" Moyers asked.

"Let me give you a musical analogy," Delbanco answered. "If I'm going to play the violin, I have to know some very concrete things. I have to know where to put my fingers, how to draw the bow, how hard to push, how quickly to draw, and so forth. To a certain degree there's a science of violin playing. But if I want to make the music really speak to you, then I have to do something that goes beyond just these mechanics. Medicine is no different from that. I've got to go beyond the technical aspects of this test and that part of your body. I've got to somehow try to understand your spirit and maybe even touch it at times."

■

Medicine also needs to make practical changes—in teaching young physicians the reality of the world outside the hospitals where they train. Some of this is happening. But when I asked the AMSA students in Boston if they had taken a class in economics, health policy, or business management, they said no. Nor is it clear that the new courses educators are teaching in empathy and ethics during the first two years are truly acting to humanize the sudden plunge into the grueling reality of the third-year clerkship or the residency.

Most important of all, we need to return to a sense of sanity, to a lessening of extremes, so that someone like Carol Tisch is able to mature and become tough enough to handle the horrors and challenges of caring for the sick, yet retain her best impulses. We need to expunge from the training anything that systematically works against what truly is the hard reality of medicine—that practicing physicians are foolish to ignore the human side, if only because they themselves are likely to be more satisfied if they understand their charges beyond hemoglobin counts and bilirubins, and embrace the real world where they will one day have to work and live.

We should also understand that there is more to medicine than the tough-guy ethos of Randy Gaines, for whom healing becomes a military operation and the physician a warrior, out for the heady thrill of launching highly skilled commando raids against disease.

Randy Gaines insists it's all for his patients, and in some ways it is, though healing is not warfare. It is not anger, bitterness, regret, or sadness. Ultimately, and most sensibly, it should be an act of deep commitment, respect—and, yes, of love.

CHAPTER 8

Do the Kind Thing First

I see no reason or need for my doctor to love me—nor would I expect him to suffer with me. I wouldn't demand a lot of my doctor's time: I just wish he would brood on my situation for perhaps five minutes, that he would give me his whole mind just once, be bonded with me for a brief space, survey my soul as well as my flesh, to get at my illness, for each man is ill in his own way.

Anatole Broyard, "Intoxicated by My Illness"

In the surgeon's amphitheater, beneath life-size portraits of surgeons long dead, the seats were arranged on a steep incline. At the bottom, closest to the speaker, sat a half-dozen revered vascular surgeons dressed in crisp white lab coats, expensive leather shoes, and silk ties. Each had his name embroidered in green thread above his left breast pocket, sewn in cursive swirls. Angling up behind them, in rigid order, were junior faculty, fellows, and residents arranged backward by year—PGY 5s, 4s, 3s, 2s and, way up top, the interns.

"Let's begin," says the speaker, a senior resident. Instantly, the buzz in the amphitheater dies down. "Our first patient is an eighty-eight-year-old male," he says, speaking without notes. The senior resident, a small, haughty man with thinning brown hair and a slight swagger in his step, ordered an intern (you could tell his ranking by his short white coat) to wheel in the patient.

"Ladies and gentlemen, Mr. Ivan Maximov," said the doctor, gesturing like P. T. Barnum to a patient I was surprised to recognize—an elderly demented man with vascular disease admitted a couple of days earlier to the medicine ward in this hospital, where I had been following an intern, Pete Nichols, during an overnight call. In pain and frightened, this old man had moaned all night, keeping up half the ward. Every so often he screamed, sounding as if he were being tortured. I was especially curious to see him here since I knew his family had been furious at the hospital's vascular surgeons when they refused to operate on their grandfather, saying he was too old and frail. I wondered if they had given permission for their revered pater to be here like this, on display.

All eyes went forward, trained on a feeble, skinny heap of a man sprawled out on a gurney, his baggy flesh and bones covered only by a thin, wrinkled white sheet Mr. Maximov had instinctively pulled upward to cover most of his face. Like a child, this essentially witless old man peered over the top of the sheet, dazed and confused by the roomful of eyes. Rolled into a dense ball and clutched tight to his chest was an orange, yellow, and white wool coverlet, a comfort from home his family had brought for him, like a baby's blanket.

"Here we have an example of an elderly man with advanced cardiovascular disease in both legs," announced the resident. "Mental status negligible, renal failure, mild myositis. . . ." He kept speaking, describing a man at the end of life, with multiple chronic and soon-to-be fatal problems. He ended his flawless presentation with the pertinent question, which I already knew the answer to: was this eighty-eight-year-old male a candidate for a bypass to restore blood flow to his ankles and feet? Without the operation, he might lose his feet.

■

From what I could gather about Ivan Maximov, he had emigrated from Russia as a young man. Arriving with very little, he had built a successful family business which he had run with his sons and grandsons until well into his eighties. When Pete Nichols had first visited him, his room was crowded with somber members of his clan— well dressed, well educated, and obviously doting on the old man.

One of Ivan's relatives was trying not to become too angry as he demanded that Pete Nichols arrange the surgery. All he could say was that it was the surgeons' call, and they had said no. Afterward, Pete told me the surgeons were right; the old man might even die on the operating table. "He's their patriarch, I guess," said Pete. "They want everything possible done. They can't face that he's dying."

In the afterglow of his perfect presentation, the resident and the entire room waited with great anticipation as the revered vascular surgeons looked at one another, deciding with nods and gestures who should deliver the answer—and seal the fate of Ivan Maximov's lower extremities.

One of them stood up. He was the youngest looking—he didn't have a single gray hair—with round, wire-rim glasses and a white coat so stiff with starch I thought it might shatter.

"Does this man speak Russian?" he asked in mock-seriousness, hearing that Max had long ago come from Russia.

"He doesn't speak," quipped the resident as everyone laughed, sitting high above this shriveled old man clasping a blanket—a man so far gone, he did not know enough to even cry.

■

For centuries, medical educators in the West have placed great importance on presenting formal case studies to groups of students with live patients on hand, even when the conditions discussed were not particularly interesting to look at, like Ivan Maximov's diseased vessels. (Ivan's legs were red and swollen; otherwise there was nothing significant in his physical appearance.) In part, this was because there were no photographs or videos to use as teaching tools, and in part because students were not routinely allowed into hospital wards to see disease unfold.

Even today, including the patient in a lecture setting can be helpful if he or she is part of the discussion and is treated with respect. Traditionally, however, patients have stood, sat, or lain mute and on exhibit as a physician-instructor pointed or jabbed, delivering the didactic lesson of the day. In the nineteenth and early twentieth centuries, instructors performed surgery in the amphitheater/classroom setting, cutting open patients like Ivan Maximov in full view of students and residents sitting in seats above. In 1875, Thomas Eakins painted a famous oil of Pennsylvania surgeon Samuel Gross, dressed in a black suit and wielding a scalpel in his bare, unsterilized hand, turning away from a bloody incision to make a point to students seated in tiers of seats, calmly taking notes. A relative of the patient, seated nearby, covers his face, unable to watch—a gesture of pain and dismay counterpoised by the cool detachment of Dr. Gross and his colleagues.

In the modern era, since the invention of photography and videos and the inclusion of trainees on the wards, the tradition of using live examples in grand rounds has become less common, particularly if the patient is unable to fully grasp the proceedings. Some programs, however, persist in parading even unknowing and demented patients for a supposedly educational experience, betraying attitudes still lurking for some in the shadows of medical science—that patients are specimens, not people; that disease is not suffering but an intellectual curiosity, like a quasar or a newly discovered species of ant.

If anyone has any doubt that this insensitivity remains imbedded in the physician culture they should read a 1994 study in *The New England Journal of Medicine* on the subject of freshly dead patients' being used for teaching purposes shortly after they expired, without asking anyone's permission. According to the report, dozens of hospitals in the United States routinely turn over patients' bodies to residents for them to practice everything from inserting tubes in tracheas to opening chests to learn heart massage. In teaching certain skills, cadavers are sometimes preferable to live patients, but not when physicians assume they have the right to use a person's body as they see fit without obtaining the proper permissions. It is even worse when live patients are treated callously in the name of education, particularly as the object of an anachronistic ritual with little modern practical value.

■

Of course, physicians are not entirely to blame for lingering manners more befitting the last century than this one. Indeed, the public has only recently begun backing off an awe-struck reverence for physicians and medical science that has, after all, produced a dizzying progression of miraculous new cures and technologies. For decades, this has meant that patients showed little interest in what happened within the walls of hospitals and research centers, assuming their physicians would behave paternalistically, and would watch out for their best interests. Most did, though this complacency also allowed medicine to perpetuate a colder, more clinical side of dealing with some patients out of the public eye.

Inevitably, however, as generations who can remember polio epidemics and diabetes without insulin pass on, and as science loses its power to dazzle us in an age of AIDs and other incurable ills, both patients and physicians are evolving away from the old lop-sided relationship. Patients these days want and sometimes demand more from their healers, while doctors, particularly young ones, increasingly want to include patients in the details of their care—both for ethical reasons and because they find a process of sharing, when possible, far more fulfilling than treating patients like mere bundles of tissue, bone, and fluids.

This new relationship lies at the core of new medical school courses on ethics and on "the doctor-patient relationship"—which is a step in the right direction, though one need spend only a few minutes following residents to see that the laudable philosophy of classroom ethics frequently fails to penetrate into the wards. Indeed, knowing that ethics is taught and rules of compassion and morality opined makes it all the more unnerving to spend time in teaching hospitals where old attitudes persist, seemingly oblivious to the passage of time. In part, this is because large urban hospitals have too long been worlds unto themselves, ivory towers where nearly everyone is either a health care specialist or very sick, and where many patients have nothing whatsoever in common with the physicians who attend to them.

To an outsider lingering on the wards, the proof accumulates in ways large and small. For starters, there remains a bemusing, pseu-doscientific nineteenth-century sensibility about how physicians in teaching hospitals refer to patients as "male" or "female" rather than men, women, and children. I once asked an intern who referred to the "eighty-seven-year-old male in 314B" if she meant a human male or some other animal. Some thirty hours into her shift, she did not find this funny. Even more curious is the habit of identifying "cases" and "conditions" instead of people—the "eighty-eight-year-old male with diseased vessels"; the "wheezer* in room 916"; or, worse, "the boxoid GOMER on the fifth floor."

More jarring for an outsider is how physicians talk about their "cases" in front of the patients, as if they weren't there. On rounds, where large clusters of doctors and students, both senior and junior, engulf the patient in a kind of bedside version of the old grand rounds, attendings quiz interns about test results, diagnoses, and what to rule out or to keep on considering—often with the patient lying inches away. I remember one woman watching this exchange

---

*Slang for anyone with asthma or congested lungs who has trouble breathing.

as she would the action in a tennis match. The attending to her left asked; "Did you rule out cocaine?" "Yes," answered the intern on the right side of the bed. "The results were negative."

"And what about the bilirubin?" Back to the left side. "Is it still too high?"

"It's at 16."

"Does that worry you?"

Patients I spoke with found this process bewildering and occasionally frightening. "I don't like it," claimed a woman in her forties whose abdominal cavity was rapidly filling with fluid, making her appear nine months pregnant. "It's like I'm not here." A few minutes earlier, a medical student had "presented" her to the chief resident and a half-dozen others on this team. It was the student's first formal "case," and he was obviously nervous. Trying to speak from memory, he kept anxiously peeking toward the notecards he clutched in his hand.

"Come over here," said the chief when the student was finished. He touched the woman's belly without asking her permission, or if it hurt her. She gazed at the doctors as wide-eyed as a child while the medical student reached out a tentative, gloved hand toward her belly. Impatiently, the chief grabbed his hand and pressed it to the woman's stomach. She winced.

"What do you feel?" asked the chief, addressing the medical student.

"It feels like, ah, ah, liquid," he stammered, instantly realizing he had said something embarrassingly obvious. His face turned red.

"So what should we be thinking here?" asked the chief.

"We're thinking TB," jumped in the intern who had been supervising the medical student, saving him from further embarrassment. "Ascites. Maybe edema."

"Or chronic Hep-B," said the medical student hopefully. He had just stolen a glance at his notes.

"Mental status?" asked the chief.

"She's alert," said the intern.

"I want this tapped," the chief said to the team, meaning he wanted a tube inserted to drain the fluid from the woman's abdomen. "And I want you to keep after it"—meaning he wanted a diagnosis as quickly as possible. Only then did he glance at the patient and mutter a thank-you before whirring around in a flurry of starch and white to march over to the next patient. The team quickly followed, with the intern shuffling through his notes, since this time *he* would be presenting the next "case" by memory.

I found the lack of everyday courtesy in such scenes disturbing—and very, very common. I can't imagine most of these physicians' treating friends or casual acquaintances this way outside the hospital. In another instance, I am perplexed as to why doctors feel it necessary to yell at virtually every patient over sixty, as if they were deaf—"MRS. JONES, DOES YOUR CHEST HURT TODAY? DID YOU URINATE OKAY?"—even when Mrs. Jones can obviously hear. Doctors and nurses also seem oblivious much of the time to waking patients at all hours, frequently to ask trivial questions, or for residents and students to repeat examinations and histories that should have been done earlier. This happens in part because residents are too busy during normal waking hours to tend to routine matters.

Likewise, trainees almost never properly identified themselves as interns, residents, and medical students. A common deceit in teaching hospitals is allowing patients to assume that medical school students are M.D.'s—calling them "doctor," though they may be years from earning their degree. Many times, when I returned to interview patients after rounds, they were only vaguely aware that they were even in a teaching hospital, or that some of the many doctors tending them were not fully trained. Most academic centers make it clear in their admission papers that a patient might be treated by residents, but this is often buried in a thicket of fine print. Some patients I met even had a hard time identifying their chief physician, particularly when the intern who admitted them moved at the end of the month to a new rotation, and another PGY1 or medical student became "their" doctor. When I told them the physician legally responsible for them was the attending who typically came around only in the morning for a brief visit, if at all, just a handful understood that he or she was their official doctor of record.

Ethicist Edmund Pellegrino, for one, is highly critical of this deep-seated insensitivity in teaching hospitals, especially the style of instruction in which crowds of white coats surround a patient in his bed. "This is the wrong way to teach," he says. "Why? Because first of all the patient is there to be healed, to be helped. He is not there as a teaching object. He may consent to be part of the teaching process, but even then, people he hasn't met before are standing around him and the teacher makes the patient the object, and you have people pawing the patient. Then you are using medical terminology. Don't kid yourself;

every word you use in front of the patient has an impact. This is bad pedagogy, bad teaching, and bad for the patient."

Of course, the best residents and attendings devote far more time to patients than these formal rounds permit. If allowed the time— sometimes a big *if*— most tell me the only way to truly master the healer's art is to go solo and repeatedly tap a patient's belly, perform an incision, or talk patients through their fears and concerns. This was the point of Osler's revolution.

Yet a barrier remains between doctor and patient, seemingly by design, as I saw some trainees taught by example to be uncivil, and that it is all right to act as if a patient isn't really there. Part of this distancing is inevitable, since physicians have to be wary about plunging *too* far into patients and disease. "What these young people see can be horrible and distressing," said Rhode Island's Ed Iannuccilli. "If you are at all compassionate, you cannot survive long in this environment without distancing yourself. And you certainly cannot operate as you must as a compassionate doctor if you allow yourself to become overwhelmed by tragedy."

Essayist Anatole Broyard, for one, found the buffers put up by his doctors baffling—and even sad—as prostate cancer slowly killed him in the early 1990s. "Physicians have been taught in medical school that they must keep the patient at a distance because there isn't time to accommodate his personality," writes Broyard in a bittersweet essay first delivered as a speech at the University of Chicago Medical School shortly after he was diagnosed, "or because if the doctor becomes *involved* in the patient's predicament, the emotional burden will be too great. As I've suggested, it doesn't take much time to make good contact, but beyond that, the emotional burden of *avoiding* the patient may be much harder on the doctor than he imagines. It may be this that sometimes makes him complain of feeling harassed. A doctor's job would be so much more interesting and satisfying if he simply let himself plunge into the patient, if he could lose his own fear of falling."

■

Since at least the time of Hippocrates, educators and philosophers have warned against physicians' losing touch with patients. "The intimacy also between physician and patient is close," opines the ancient Greek corpus that bears Hippocrates' name, adding that a hard edge is to be avoided, "for harshness is taken to mean arrogance and unkindness." Likewise, one of the most frequently quoted quips of William Osler is: "Do the kind thing and do it first." Lately, research has begun to suggest that direct time spent interacting with patients and ministering to their emotional needs can even improve outcomes, and possibly lower costs. Consider the following:

- At the University of Minnesota, out of a hundred patients receiving bone marrow transplants for leukemia, researchers found that over half who felt they had strong emotional support from family and physicians survived the transplants for at least two years. Only 20 percent survived among those who said they had little support.
- In New York and Chicago, a study jointly conducted by Mt. Sinai Hospital and Northwestern University Medical School found that elderly patients admitted for hip fractures were discharged an average of two days sooner when they were provided mental health care and counseling, compared to patients given the usual standard of care just for their fractures. The shorter stays saved the hospital $178,572, less a psychiatric tab of $21,760.
- In yet another study, 122 men were rated as feeling optimistic or pessimistic at the time of suffering a heart attack. Eight years later, their state of mind ended up being a better predictor of death by heart attack than damage to the heart after the earlier attack, arterial blockage, cholesterol levels, or blood pressure.

This hardly means that a patient's emotional state outweighs purely biological problems, or that "doing the kind thing first" should replace scientific medical care. But according to Dr. James Strain, the lead author of the study on elderly patients with hip fractures; "Physicians absolutely should take their patients' emotional state into account when they treat them for medical problems."

Of course, these studies and others like them are merely another case of medical science's needing quantifiable data to draw a conclusion that is intuitively obvious. Hippocrates knew what researchers at Mt. Sinai, Northwestern, and the University of Minnesota had to prove scientifically: that "for some patients, though conscious that their condition is perilous, recover their health simply through their contentment with the goodness of the physician."

■

This situation resonates with irony. For inasmuch as there is a movement in the United States toward more empathy and patient rights, it's occurring in direct opposition to what physician-scientists have spent most of this century trying to instill: the notion that what patients have to say about their illness is less important than the science, and sometimes irrelevant to a purely scientific inquiry, if the patient is distraught or overly emotional. As recently as 1985, an editorial in *The New England Journal of Medicine* dismissed the idea that emotions play any significant role in treating disease, calling such ideas "largely folklore."

This dismissal has its roots in the steep ascendancy of science during the past century—what one can see, feel, and measure—which replaced what had been for centuries a physician's heavy reliance on a patient's own version of his or her illness. In fact, before the stethoscope and subsequent devices allowed physicians to peek inside the body and measure critical functions, the patient history—plus whatever manifestations of disease appeared on the body's surface—was all a physician had to go by. Sometimes, well-known physicians would not even physically see patients, who would write from outlying areas or distant cities describing their illnesses. The doctor would then write back a diagnosis and suggest a cure.

The new scientist-physicians of Osler's era considered these descriptive examinations to be impressionistic, fallible, and far less important than, say, the number of times per minute an asthmatic took a breath, or the diameter of an incontinent man's kidney. Indeed, anyone who has heard patients describe their problems can agree that this is hardly an exact science. Even when not comatose, sedated, or delirious with fever, patients are not always honest or objective—which is to be expected from ill and frightened people. "Patients lie all the time," said one surgical intern. This is particularly true, he noted, when illicit drugs or sex are involved, or a patient does not want to admit to himself that he's ill.

But it's also true that contemporary medicine, with its Magnetic

Resonance Imagers and techniques to isolate cancer-causing genes, seems to have become so dependent on technology that in many cases it has thrown out the wisdom of previous generations along with what was truly "folklore." In part, this stems from the transformation launched by Osler and his generation, who intended not only to expunge subjectivity in medicine but also to rid the United States of a medical education system steeped in empiricism, pseudoscience, and outright quackery. The culmination of this effort for medical education came in 1910, when a young educator named Abraham Flexner wrote a scathing critique of medical schools and their lack of attention to science. Flexner's report, *Medical Education in the U.S. and Canada*, triggered the closing of dozens of fly-by-night medical schools and encouraged a massive retrofitting of those still open.

Like so many other trends in medicine that have proved useful in the past, however, Osler's and Flexner's imperative has overshot the mark. Even Flexner, who lived until 1960, understood the downside of a profession that became too obsessed with science at the expense of the core reason why physicians exist—to minister to the ill. "Now science," he wrote in 1930, "while widening our vision, increasing our satisfactions and solving our problems, brings with it dangers peculiarly its own. We can become so infatuated with progress in knowledge and control—both of which I have unstintingly emphasized—that we lose our perspective, lose our historic sense, lose a philosophic outlook, lose sight of relative cultural values."

In another treatise, Flexner accused educators of "a curious mis-apprehension" of his ideas, saying it was never his intent for science to squeeze out what he called "medical humanism" and a "sensitivity to human suffering." Writing in the forties, Flexner even predicted a time when the public would distrust scientific medicine, if physicians continued to deny moral challenges posed by new technologies. "In the modern university," he wrote, "the more vigorously science is prosecuted, the more acute the need that society [places on us to] be held accountable . . . Philosophers and critics, therefore, gain in importance as science makes life more complex—more rational in some ways, more irrational in others."

Osler, who believed more than anything in reasonableness, would probably be appalled at what has happened. Medicine, he said, should embrace what he called "the cold logic" of science, but not at the expense of humaneness. Physicians, he believed, should "recognize the true poetry of life—the poetry of the commonplace, of the ordinary man, of the plain, toil-worn woman, with their loves and their joys, their sorrows and their griefs." Like Anatole Broyard, Osler advocated that physicians should sometimes even laugh. "Illness is not all tragedy," wrote Broyard, the patient. "Much of it is funny." In 1905, Osler the physician declared to medical students in Canada: "The comedy, too, of life will be spread before you, and nobody laughs more often than the doctor."

Of course, not all physicians think this way, particularly those who believe only that "the cold logic" of science is truly valid in the practice of medicine. Even those doctors who would like to be more empathetic to their patients typically react skeptically to talk about poetry and plunging into one's patient. In fact, according to ethicist Edmund Pellegrino, a fundamental tension exists in medicine between science and the humanities—which he says "are, and always will remain, two different ways of looking at reality, each with its own perspective, method, and rules of evidence." Yet this hardly means that science is incompatible with humanism, says Pellegrino. "The number of scientists with humane interests is impressive," he writes, maintaining that the well-versed physician knows how to apply the two in unison and in appropriate proportions.

At the risk of sounding hopelessly mired in "touchy-feely," humanistic nonsense, I am forced to agree with Broyard, Osler, and Pellegrino: that it's critical for physicians—scientists and humanists alike—to understand, or at least to appreciate, the difference between laughter and tragedy, science and poetry. I don't want to belabor this point, since those who need things quantified are already shaking their heads and thinking this is all high and mighty fluff. Yet I think it remains unfortunate that as recently as 1986, according to a survey of physicians who attended three eastern colleges, only 14 percent had earned degrees in the humanities—which may partly explain why nonscience majors in medical school are known, not always fondly, as "poets." Since 1986, after a concerted effort, medical schools have managed to enroll more "poets."* Perhaps as time goes on, their impact will be more profoundly felt.

---

*The AMSA students in Boston told me about "nontraditional students" at Tufts and Pittsburgh, including "Bob the cop," a fellow student who had been a policeman for nine years in Washington, D.C.; "Jenny," who did missionary work in India; and a forty-one-year-old woman who once worked welding together nuclear submarines for the navy.

■

This is not to say that medical science, and the hard sort of pragmatism that Broyard decries, is not terribly useful—particularly when one's bedside manner is irrelevant to a patient who will die without the skill of a scientist, and the touch not of a human hand but of a scalpel, arthroscope, or specialized drug. The vast majority of patients, however, are *not* in acute distress. A percentage I often hear is that 90 percent of all patients seen by the nation's 650,000 physicians are not dying, not having heart attacks, and not in an immediate crisis.

Yet medicine continues to heavily tilt the residency toward the 10 percent of patients who are most ill, plunging trainees into a world of almost constant crisis, where the number of tasks becomes so overwhelming that it should come as no surprise that residents have little time for anything but science, which by necessity must come first. "There is no time to think about anything but what's happening with Mr. Smith's fluids, or Mrs. Smith's arrhythmia," said a young Seattle attending who majored in religion and history, "so you fall back on the mechanisms of care, and diagnosis, and the ABCs of the science. Everything becomes a crisis because of lack of time, whether it's a real crisis or not."

"This crisis mentality is, I think, mostly a matter of poor planning these days," said a surgical chief resident in New York City, "because most really sick people today, even in a hospital, don't die. In years past, it was more of a crapshoot, a matter of busting butt to get to everyone quick or they would die. The overwhelming urgency is no longer there, because most people aren't going to die in the next five minutes. We can stablize them and keep them alive for a long time. Most people, in fact, don't die in hospitals but survive to go home—which is different from fifty or a hundred years ago."

Recently, with the advent of managed care and the economic demand for primary care doctors to act as patient "gatekeepers," residency programs have added more rotations in outpatient clinics and private physicians' offices. The idea here is not only to train "gatekeepers" but also to move trainees out of the rarefied world of hospitals and into the community where most doctors actually practice. Yet even in primary care programs, residents still spend the bulk of their time inside the walls of the hospital. At one facil-

ity I studied, which considers itself progressive, pediatricians appor-
tion fully one-sixth of their three years in the Neonatal Intensive
Care Unit, a high-tech domain few of these trainees will enter again
after they finish. Of course, they need to be exposed to the workings
of the NICU. But why a total of six months?

For many trainees, the emphasis on scientific medicine
inevitably feeds into technology's natural allure, particularly for the
majority of physicians who have been scientists all along. Indeed,
technology can be breathtaking when a young scientist (or poet)
begins to master machines and protocols that seem like something
out of science fiction—and can also produce far more dramatic and
quantifiable results than a mere touch or a kind word.

"High tech is like the new toys on the block," a young primary care
attending at Boston's Beth Israel Hospital told me, a year after finishing her residency. "We're like fresh kids. We want to play with just the
toys. This can be very seductive. But then some of us have said, Wait
a minute here, we didn't go to medical school to play with
machines, and drips, and to give you this much lidocaine and
neosynephrine, and basically run a human lab. For me, I went to medical school to be connected to human suffering, to make things better."

I asked her if her training as a medical student had prepared her for
the nonscience part of her job. "That's not the emphasis," she said.
"Everything in the early training, from premed to late in medical
school, is based on a reward system for getting the answers right on a
test. This doesn't help much when you're dealing with the human
problems. I've found that the nuts and bolts of medicine, the basic science—how to resuscitate, how to support someone so they can
breathe—this you can learn to do almost like a technician, and
without thinking this is somebody's father, and there are kids there
crying in the waiting room worried if Dad will live or die. But it's having to tell someone they have AIDS, or a young woman she has
breast cancer, these are where the training falls down."

Young physicians tell me they are taught these skills only if they
are lucky enough to have instructors who see beyond the machines.
"It's no wonder we are so biased toward science," the Beth Israel
attending claimed. "We are taught almost exclusively by scientists,
Ph.D.'s, and bench M.D.'s who leave their labs to attend on the
wards, or give lectures, only with great reluctance." It's hardly surprising, then, that young doctors immersed in the culture of the

machine sometimes find themselves behaving like machines themselves, toiling endless hours to complete technical tasks as if sleep didn't matter, or family, or their own health.

I wonder if this quest to be a machine—to follow the "cold logic" of Osler's science, with art and charity at best a distant second and third place—contributed to the suffering of Mary Allen during Jim Stern's thirty-one-hour shift. What if Stern had spent eight minutes with Mary and her family for every one minute writing notes and analyzing tests, instead of the opposite? The scientific outcome—death—would have been the same. But I suspect the emotional outcome would have been much improved for doctor, patient, and family.

■

In 1992, William Hurt played Jack McKee, M.D., in *The Doctor*, a film version of Dr. Edward Rosenbaum's book, *A Taste of My Own Medicine*. A Hollywood stereotype of a callous, wisecracking heart surgeon who learns empathy after his own bout with disease, McKee at first behaves like a monster of haughtiness to his patients. With one woman in her forties, recovering from open heart surgery, he responds to concerns about her chest scar by telling her not to worry, because she looks like a *Playboy* centerfold. "And you have the staple marks to prove it," he says, snickering.

Of course, this patient and all the others mistreated by McKee get their payback when their doctor contracts throat cancer and is treated to his own dose of this movie's version of a cold, heartless system. The film then ends with a marvelous teaching scene, where the newly compassionate McKee takes a band of greenhorn residents and orders them into examination rooms to don hospital gowns.

"Doctors," says McKee as this particularly handsome stable of interns, direct from central casting, stand awkwardly in their flimsy, all-too-revealing frocks, "you have spent a lot of time learning the Latin names for diseases your patients might have. Now it's time to learn something simpler about them. Patients have their own names." He tacks up the name of each resident on the door of a vacant patient room, minus the "M.D." "They feel frightened, embarrassed, and vulnerable. And they feel sick. Most of all, they want to get better. Because of that, they put their lives in our hands. I could try to explain what that means until I'm blue in the face. But you know something, it wouldn't mean a thing. It sure as hell never did to me. So for the next seventy-two hours, you'll each be allocated a particular disease. You'll sleep in hospital beds, eat hospital food, and you'll be given all the appropriate tests." He says this as a half-dozen nurses wheel in drug carts, I.V.'s on poles, and various nasty looking devices and machines.

"You are no longer doctors," he says, moving toward the door of the ward to leave, "you're hospital patients." As he opens the door, they stare at him in shock.

"So good luck. I'll see you on my rounds."

Though this movie leaves none of its themes to the imagination—the doctor is bad, gets his own, becomes good—it does highlight the paradox at the core of what can go wrong between doctor and patient, between medical science and humanism; that it is difficult for a healer to fully understand and to feel compassion for a condition they have never known. But can compassion be taught to medical trainees in a meaningful way? This is not an idle question. For centuries, philosophers have debated whether or not compassion—formerly known as charity—can be learned, or whether one is either born with it, or not.

William Osler, for one, had doubts about the teachability of certain behavioral attributes, describing "imperturbability," for instance, as "largely a bodily endowment" that some people will never acquire, "owing to congenital defects." Yet Osler also believed that education and practice could still "do much." Edmund Pellegrino agrees, submitting that if Abraham Flexner were writing a report on medical education today, he would rail against the lack of humanities in today's curriculum as loudly as he did about the scientific deficiencies in 1910.

Of course, these days the issue has become somewhat moot, given a rising demand by patients that physicians pay more attention to their emotional needs—and even, on occasion, "plunge into them," as Anatole Broyard suggested. As I have mentioned, this has happened in part because technology is providing medicine with far more choices that patients should participate in, and want to. Indeed, the burgeoning if belated consumer movement is finally engulfing medicine, with the promise that colonoscopies will soon be scrutinized for quality and cost like mini-vans, can openers, and VCRs.

"Today's sensibilities are more informed by consumers than they were in the old days," says Tom Delbanco. "Our industry has been slow to come to that, that you should listen to the customer." This is more evident than ever as HMOs talk about "quality assurance," and states such as Pennsylvania and New York begin to publish consumer ratings of hospitals' and physicians' mortality rates. Before long, I have no doubt that *Consumer Reports* will be listing hospitals and procedures, and rating them with red and black circles half full, full, and empty according to who performs the best CABG, and which doctor can best set a broken toe.

■

The changing dynamic between doctors and patients has not been missed by most medical schools. When I perused the current handbook describing curricula at each school, virtually every one of them offered elective courses in ethics, the history of medicine, literature and medicine, or patient interaction—or combinations of all four. About two-thirds offered required courses in ethics in the first two years, taught right alongside neurology, immunology, and pharmacology.

The problem is that these courses are sometimes not taken as seriously as they should be by educators or students, with some programs shoe-horning a few hours of ethics into a still massive regimen of science and physiology. Others spend more time, though most any student will tell you that given a choice between studying the liver and the four principles of justice in patient care, the liver wins.

Far worse is what happens to the lessons in empathy and concern for the patient's rights and humanity when medical students suddenly find themselves on the wards in their third-year clerkships, or later, when they plunge into their internships. Take the case of Ivan Maximov and the impact of his ordeal on the interns and medical students sitting far up on the amphitheater's incline. What were they to think as they watched the revered, wisecracking surgeons making fun of this frail old man?

Presumably, in medical school, they were taught the concept of patient autonomy, defined in a widely used ethics textbook as follows:

> To respect an autonomous agent is, at a minimum, to acknowledge that person's right to hold views, to make

choices, and to take actions based on personal values and beliefs. Such respect involves respectful *action*, not merely a respectful attitude.

This definition, or one like it, is probably on every medical ethics final exam in every medical school that teaches the subject. Yet it's clear whom the interns in that amphitheater, under the steady gaze of local giants in their field, will believe.

Likewise, listening to Carol Tisch talk about the Little Hitlers and the ethical lapses in her training, it appears that some residents experience wide gaps between what they see and experience, and what their first-year ethics block taught them. "As wonderful and innovative as ethics classes can be," says medical anthropologist and physician counselor John-Henry Pfifferling, who has closely studied physician training, "I don't think it has much impact after medical school. It comes up now and then in the neonatal intensive care unit, and sometimes in a difficult end-of-life situation, but you really get little of it in the clinical trenches. And with that nonexposure, the residents see what's happening around them, and emulate it. If your senior resident and attendings are compassionate, you will be, because that's what's expected. But if they aren't, you learn to ignore it."

Add fatigue, overwork, and undue stress to the equation, and you beget situations like Mary Allen's and countless others, where a compassionate young physician was ready and willing to do the right thing—but was too busy and pressured to grasp what this was, or to implement it. This suggests yet another crucial dilemma that brings us back to the great flaw in the classic plunge-in method: how can we expect a trainee to know ethics if we simply let him or her loose with only a few definitions from a book learned two or three years earlier?

Just as it seems like a lot to ask neophyte interns to start a central line by themselves, having done only one or two before, it seems a stretch to expect residents to know how to practice good ethics without some formal guidance or example "in the trenches." Attendings such as Jennifer Jeremiah and Bill Frishman prove compassion can be compatible with good medicine—and daily stress this point to their residents. Some residencies are also running an ongoing ethics curriculum in the wards. One of these is headed by Georgetown's Edmund Pellegrino, whose Center for Clinical Bioethics always has an ethicist on call to answer ethical questions that arise in the hospital. The day I visited Pellegrino, he showed me his department's "ethics" beeper. "I'm called all the time," he says, adding that theoretic ethics is fine, but only if you find a way to apply it clinically. At Rhode Island Hospital, Brown University philosopher Dan Brock visits medicine wards for scheduled ethics rounds to hash out real-life dilemmas with residents. "The teaching has a very practical context to it," says Brock, "because it's framed around a case that's selected by the residents, an actual case that's usually on the service at the time. We are not trying to create junior bioethicists or junior philosophers. What we are trying to do is use the actual ethical issues that arise for physicians as part of training."

Issues covered by Brock range from when to forgo life support to whether or not it's ethical to eat free pizza provided by pharmaceutical companies trying to get doctors to use their name-brand drugs. Most hospitals also convene ethics panels (and risk-management committees) to decide ethical dilemmas that may bring on legal action, or that involve differences of opinion among physicians and/or physicians and families regarding specific cases.

Still, a great deal slips through the cracks.

One poignant ethical lapse that was never the subject of ethics rounds—it was considered just one of those things—sticks in my mind from the spring of 1993. It involves an HIV-positive thirty-two-year-old man who was operated on to have fluid drained from around his heart, only to have the surgical intern in charge put off for almost a week removing a drainage tube the patient no longer needed, despite the fact he faced a high risk of infection from a weakened immune system.

"I don't think they realize that I'm HIV positive," said Bob Zapita, a soft-spoken man with a Vandyke beard. He caught HIV while shooting up cocaine a couple of years earlier with an infected needle. By "they" he meant the surgeons, who were consulting on a case being managed by the medicine residents. "To leave this thing in longer than needed is asking for trouble," says Zapita. "It's just going to mean something else is going to happen, pneumonia or something. I'm still healthy, but who knows how long that will last? I want to fight this thing myself."

The reasons the surgical intern didn't take out the tube each day varied; he was either too busy to walk over to the medicine ward, or he was in the O.R. One night when the medicine intern called to demand he remove the tube, the surgical intern told her he needed to have his attending's permission—but the attending was at home, he said, and the intern refused to disturb him.

Meanwhile, Zapita sat stoically in a chair beside his bed, looking out at the sky and smiling sadly as the medicine intern kept promising the tube would come out. "She's a good doctor," he said. "But she just doesn't seem to have the authority to do what she says. I know it bugs the hell out of her. I'm grateful for that."

■

In the end, compassion—and empathy, charity, kindness, humanism, or whatever word one wants to use—remains a slippery, difficult concept to grasp, yet anyone who has felt the touch of a healer, or a loved one, at a moment of crisis knows it is real. Perhaps not as real as the hard surface of a scalpel when a hernia needs to be repaired, but nonetheless a critical part of healing.

"I think the doctor-patient relationship is a very important relationship," says Tom Delbanco, "and I think it might become more important if we can do it right, because there are so few human anchors left to us, and we've become so depersonalized, with faxes and so forth. So we lust for human contact. You go to a movie that makes you cry. And you hope you can kiss your wife in the dark and quiet in a romantic atmosphere instead of in front of your office, or, if you're a doctor, in front of an operating room. And you hope that your doctor will be someone who reaches out and even puts his or her arm around you, and says it's going to be all right. I think we all need that more rather than less. With the little more compassion that's left in society, I hope doctors can provide some of that. It's important medicine. It would be tragic if we fall prey to these almost inexorable forces that move us along with everyone else."

This ideal, though, remains elusive for now, as evidenced by what happened to Ivan Maximov that morning in the amphitheater. Certainly, no one there was reaching out to him, or putting their arms around him. Instead, one of the respected vascular surgeons, when asked by the residents if they should operate, stepped up to the gurney and simply tucked the sheet under Ivan's emaciated feet—to lots of snickering—indicating he saw no reason to bother with such a pathetic old man, who was going to die anyway.

CHAPTER 9

An Intern Forever

*. . . the internship, in the course of years, [has] accumu-
lated a number of defects which [have] become fixed by
virtue of their long existence.*

Statement from the Interne Council of America, 1940

■

For over a decade, Sidney Zion has raged against medicine. A
loud, cigar-smoking New Yorker, Zion is currently a columnist
for the *Daily News;* a graduate of Yale Law School, former federal
prosecutor, magazine publisher, crime thriller novelist, Manhattan
restaurateur, biographer of Roy Cohn, and one-time legal reporter
for the *New York Times.* A round-jowled curmudgeon who is turning white-haired at sixty-one, he remains as formidable looking as
Sidney Greenstreet in *Casablanca,* crossed with the street smarts
and feistiness of an old-fashioned union boss or crusading newspa-
perman, and with a mercurial charm all his own.

According to a reporter friend of mine, a former New York state
health commissioner once said that it was a bad idea to anger Sidney Zion. Shortly after the tragic and unexpected death of his eighteen-year-old daughter, Libby, organized medicine found out why.

■

Sidney Zion's crusade began with a phone call at 7:45 A.M. on
Monday, March 5, 1984, when the Zion family doctor, Raymond
Sherman, rang him from the New York Hospital/Cornell University Medical Center. Sidney and his wife, Elsa, had taken Libby
there at 11:40 the night before, where she was admitted with a high
fever, severe dehydration, and bouts of near uncontrollable shaking
for reasons that to this day remain a mystery.

Sidney later testified during the civil suit he brought against
Sherman, three former residents, and New York Hospital that he was

sure Sherman was calling him to say Libby was okay, and that he and Elsa could come pick her up. Instead, Zion says that Sherman told him: " 'It's real bad. You have to get over here.' So I went to the bathroom to splash water on my face," Zion recalled on the stand. A moment later, the phone rang again. This time it was the intern in charge of Libby calling. As Sidney walked back in the room, he heard his wife pose a question that still haunts them both.

"Are you trying to tell me my daughter is dead?" Elsa asked. On the other end of the phone, Luise Weinstein, a PGY1 at New York Hospital, answered "Yes."

Zion says the last time he saw his daughter alive was in a four-person ward room on the fifth floor of the Payson Pavilion at New York Hospital, on Manhattan's Upper East Side. After staying with Libby until about 2:45 that morning the Zions went home, after the residents assured them that Libby would be all right. During his trial Zion dramatically recalled that last moment. "I went in to see her, and the last thing she said to me was: 'Shloft gezunt.' " He paused for a moment, fighting back a sob. "That's Yiddish," he said softly. "For 'sleep well, Daddy.' "

After Elsa—a former publishing executive who was as subdued at the trial as Sidney was emotive and public—delivered the news, Sidney says he immediately called Sherman back. "I said: 'Ray, what happened? I can't believe I left her! I feel like jumping out a window.' He said: 'Don't say that. There's nothing we could have done. If we'd had the ten best doctors in the world, there was nothing we could have done.' "

Several weeks later, says Zion, Ray Sherman telephoned again to tell him Libby's death may have been caused by the interaction of two drugs that should not be given together: Nardil, a powerful antidepressant Libby was taking at the time as prescribed by her psychiatrist, and Demerol, a painkiller that Libby's residents mistakenly gave her, believing it would ease her shaking fits. "He said it was a fluke," Zion remembers Sherman telling him, that the residents "had given Libby Demerol when she was on Nardil.

" 'But Ray,' " Zion says he answered, " 'I hear they tied her down and left her alone.' "

Zion was referring to the fact that intern Luise Weinstein was working on another floor, Payson three, between 3:30 A.M. and Libby's code at about 6:40 A.M., and never returned to check on her—despite two or three calls from Libby's nurses asking her to come and examine a patient they described as highly agitated, and getting worse. She kept rising from her bed, said the nurses. At one point, before Weinstein left, she had ripped out the I.V.'s inserted into her arm. By phone, Luise Weinstein ordered the nurses to put Libby in a "posey jacket," something like a corset that attaches to the bed. Later, the nurses put a wildly thrashing Libby in a four-point restraint.

Sherman does not recall using the word "fluke" or discussing restraints during this call. But he did apparently mention cocaine— which later became a major thrust of the hospital and doctors' defense, with their lawyers claiming that Libby may have taken cocaine before coming to the hospital. An illicit dose, they insisted in the trial, was possibly the cause of her erratic behavior, and even her death. " 'I just want you to know they're talking about this,' " Zion recalls Sherman telling him during this call, which Zion says came on Father's Day 1984, three months after Libby's death. Zion dismissed the idea as outrageous, a response he has not deviated from for over a decade.

According to the New York County Medical Examiner, blood collected by the hospital before Libby's death came out positive for cocaine in one test, and negative in another, a contradiction that pitted experts for both sides in the trial against one another. On the Zion side, their expert argued that the "positive" was probably false, since Libby's blood was diluted by a culture medium that may have contained impurities, a claim the hospital's experts disputed. Libby's urine also came out negative for cocaine, though a swab presumably taken from her nose came out positive for benzoylecgonine, a substance cocaine breaks down into after a few hours. This swab material, however, was too minute to verify the positive outcome. To further add to the confusion, blood and urine taken and tested after Libby died came out negative for cocaine.

Officially, the medical examiner determined that Libby Zion's cause of death was "acute pneumonitis," a nonspecific term that means a sudden inflammation of the lungs. The examiner also concluded that Libby died of a very high fever and "sudden collapse" soon after receiving injections of Demerol and Haldol "while in restraint for toxic agitation." Later, some experts and physicians speculated that Libby Zion died of a massive bacterial infection, or possibly from toxic shock syndrome caused by an influenza A virus, which reportedly is the "favorite cause of death" for Dr. R. Gordon Douglass, Jr., Physician-in-chief at New York Hospital. Others claimed it was a lethal mix of Nardil and Demerol, or cocaine, or other unknown substances Libby might have ingested.

Despite the confusing evidence, the hospital has long claimed that cocaine played a significant role in Libby Zion's death, producing in the civil trial several expert witnesses who said Libby's behavior the night she died was consistent with a bad reaction to cocaine, and that some of the autopsy tests at least hint she may have taken this drug before coming to the hospital. Evidence presented by the defense in pre-trial motions, and compiled in a recent book by author Natalie Robins about the Zion case, also suggest that Libby had a history of drug use, and may have taken cocaine as a teenager. None of this, however, definitively proves Libby Zion took cocaine that Saturday night in 1984.

"I'm not saying Libby never took drugs," says Zion. But he remains adamant that his daughter did not consume cocaine the night of March 4. In the trial he and his expert witnesses claimed that Libby died from other causes, with a toxic reaction between Nardil and Demerol heading the list.

More to the point, however, is the fact that Libby's doctors suspected she had illicit drugs on board when she arrived at the hospital—and said so on her chart, listing this among several other possible diagnoses they planned to investigate. Weinstein wrote in her admission note: "The possibility of a drug withdrawal situation is also a consideration." Oddly, this point was not pursued by the Zion side in the trial, though a suspicion of drug use surely should have triggered the usual tests to confirm or negate this possibility. If it had, and she *was* suffering a bad reaction to cocaine, this might have changed the course of her treatment.

The residents—Greg Stone and Luise Weinstein—testified that they did not pursue the drug hypothesis because Libby three times denied taking anything illicit. But patients frequently lie about taking illegal drugs, according to virtually every doctor I asked. Libby also was disoriented enough for the R2 that night, Greg Stone, to describe her as having "hysterical symptoms" in her chart. Physicians I consulted about this case, who informally studied Zion's medical records, were surprised that the residents did not run a routine "tox screen"—a test for drugs—to rule out cocaine. They also suggested that if the residents suspected a bacterial infection, they could have started Zion on a regimen of antibiotics—again, a standard precaution when a patient presents with a high temperature and white blood cell count. In Libby's case, the count was 18,200 (normal is 8,000 to 12,000), with a distribution of white blood cells that at least suggests a bacterial infection, according to physicians that I consulted.

Apparently, Weinstein and Stone believed Libby was stable enough to wait until the morning to run more tests, and to formulate a more definitive diagnosis. Talking to Stone by phone from his home, Dr. Sherman agreed with the residents' basic plan for Libby Zion.

Still, one of the many puzzles in this case is why the residents failed to perform a few simple, routine steps toward treating Zion's condition. This is in fact the crux of the dispute: Whether this was a lapse in judgment by inexperienced residents, a breakdown in hospital procedures, or a situation where protocol *was* followed, but still resulted in a death many believe should not have happened. The doctors involved continue to insist that they did nothing wrong. Whatever the truth, a nagging sense lingers that Libby Zion was not as well cared for that night as she might have been.

■

From the beginning, Sidney Zion says he was skeptical of the doctors' account of Libby's death. Never a man to believe anything at face value, Zion and a lawyer he retained began poking around, growing suspicious as hired physician-experts reviewed Libby's chart and other records. They claimed that her care had been slipshod, and that errors, not disease, had killed her. In June of 1985, fifteen months after Libby's death, Zion filed suit against the hospital as well as Sherman, Stone, Weinstein, and Maurice Leonard, the R2 who first saw her in the E.R. Meanwhile, Zion had contacted Manhattan District Attorney Robert Morgenthau, convincing the D.A.'s office to bring up charges to a grand jury for possible criminal indictment.

Morgenthau's grand jury met over a period of six months, from May to November 1985. They found no grounds for criminal indictment, but did issue the lengthy and highly unusual statement I quoted from earlier, castigating the residency system at New York Hospital and elsewhere in the state. After listening to twenty-two witnesses provided by both sides, the jurors claimed that the "medically deficient care and treatment in this case"—which included lack of supervision and overworked residents—was "systemic" and posed a grave potential danger to patients.

Dated December 31, 1986, and signed by Carol Berkman, justice of the New York Supreme Court, this report hit medicine like a tsunami, prompting one prominent medical journal to declare that what was delivered up on New Year's Eve 1985 was "an indictment of American graduate medical education." The public outcry in response to the grand jury report led to the Bell Commission and its recommendations in 1987, and the enactment of the Bell Regulations in 1989—a rapid-fire progression that shook medical education to its core and seemed destined at the time to radically alter the way physicians were trained in the United States.

Throughout this period Sidney Zion dug in and did battle. He went to the press, tapped connections, and ranted and railed to anyone who would listen, launching as a result of his grief and anger a campaign to reform residencies—and to clear the name of his daughter on the issue of cocaine.

■

On a sweltering July day in mid-Manhattan, eleven years and four months after Libby Zion died, I met Sidney Zion at Gallagher's Steak House on Broadway. A famous speakeasy in the twenties, Gallagher's remains a classic Old New York throwback where a mix of mostly graying theater-district lawyers, producers, writers, and the occasional playwright and Broadway actor convene for martinis, cigars, and unabashed feasts of red meat. Here longtime barkeeps serve up cocktails for regulars. When I arrived, smoke hung in the air. The walls were paneled in dark polished wood, decorated with photographs of mostly forgotten celebrities from the twenties and thirties—stage stars, producers, sports figures, gamblers, politicians, and a gangster or two. Into this world strides Sidney Zion in a seersucker suit, his cheeks pink from the heat outside. He's welcomed by a maitre d' who knows him well, and a barkeep who automatically prepares a martini for a customer who has been coming here for forty years.

A few months earlier, I had met Zion at Gallagher's on the eve of the civil trial he initiated against those he says killed his daughter. Almost eleven years after Libby's death, the trial started on November 10, 1994—after being delayed for years by legal manuevers from both sides, and by Zion's refusal to forgo a public trial and accept a settlement. At Bertrand Bell's request, both sides also had delayed to allow Bell's committee to conduct hearings without the distraction of a high-profile malpractice trial.

Standing at the bar at Gallagher's, Zion was ecstatic on the eve of his long-awaited day in court. "This time, believe me, they are going to burn," he said in his low, rumbling voice, loud enough so half the restaurant could hear what seemed at times a live version of the once larger-than-life characters in the photographs on the wall. These included political boss "Diamond Jim" Brady, socialite Damon Runyon, Babe Ruth, and dozens more.

"New York Hospital and all of those doctors will be on national television and the world will see what they do," said Zion. "They run a charnel house as a hospital. They've got an outhouse as a hospital. That's what they do. And now this will all come out. And I hope it will increase public awareness so that when you walk into a hospital you are not going to be destroyed. You are supposed to be helped and not by amateur kids who don't know anything."

As it turned out, the trial was not the big, splashy media event it might have been in the late eighties. With the Zion case now an old and familiar story, even the *New York Times*, Zion's old paper, ran only a few brief articles about the trial, most buried in the Metro section—although they did print a high-profile editorial on the Zion legacy soon after the verdict. Sidney Zion's current paper, the *Daily News*, twice gave the trial front-page tabloid treatment, and *People* ran a feature. Network television did not closely cover the trial, although NBC's *Dateline* broadcast a primetime retelling of the trial in the fall of 1995. Court TV broadcast long portions of the procedings until breaking off in January 1995 to cover the O. J. Simpson murder trial in Los Angeles.

The media's lukewarm response came partly as a response to what happened when the six jurors delivered their verdict on February 6. Indeed, to the surprise of many observers, they found against the Zion family on all but a few counts; they also said no to punitive damages, and to the millions of dollars Zion had long sought to punish the doctors and the hospital. Such an award also might have forced other residency programs to rethink their own curricula to avoid similar suits. Instead, the Zion family prevailed on only nine of forty-one counts, which ranged from whether or not Ray Sherman departed "from accepted medical practice by not going to New York Hospital to evaluate and treat Libby Zion" to whether or not resident Greg Stone departed "from accepted medical practice with respect to the chest X ray ordered for Libby Zion." Out of the nine verdicts for the plaintiff, the jury decided that only six contributed to Libby Zion's "pain and suffering or death."

Essentially, the jury did not believe that the hospital or the doctors had significantly deviated from acceptable medical practice at the time, except in the matter of the Demerol, which they found the three doctors guilty of administering to Libby, despite being contraindicated for patients taking Nardil. In Sherman's case, they didn't believe his claim of ignorance about the Demerol, apparently accepting resident Greg Stone's contention that he informed Sherman about giving Libby this drug during a phone call that night. Sherman has denied that Stone ever said this. The jury also found that Luise Weinstein had contributed to Libby's outcome by (1) failing to respond to calls by nurses asking her to tend to Libby in the three hours before her death, and (2) failing to provide "cool soaks/compress" when Libby's temperature began climbing to dangerous levels.

The jury virtually exonerated New York Hospital and its residency system in place in 1984, deciding in their favor on the matters of fatigue and supervision by dismissing both as factors that contributed to Libby Zion's death. This repudiated the 1986 grand jury's findings—though the 1995 jury had a much more narrow purview in terms of the facts and witnesses they were allowed to consider.

The panel of jurors did find the hospital had overworked Luise Weinstein, giving her too many patients to care for—a total of over forty she was cross-covering that night. This verdict was a bit odd, however, given that Weinstein's patient load was never a significant issue at the trial. Nor was this load outside the norm for 1984—or, in some places, for today. As I pointed out earlier, Weinstein was not kept away by patients in acute crisis, though she had one admission during this period. Most of the time she was apparently writing notes and taking care of routine patient matters on Payson three.

The jury's treatment of New York Hospital also differed significantly from a state finding in 1987 that the hospital had violated certain health code provisions, including the restraining of a patient without a physician's approval. The hospital, claiming they did not want to drag out appeals that might delay state approval of construction permits, agreed at the time to pay a $13,000 fine as part of a settlement in which they did not admit guilt.

But what surprised Sidney Zion and his supporters the most was the jury's "yes" verdict to the question: "Did Libby Zion ingest cocaine on March 4, 1984?" The six panelists also found that cocaine had contributed to Libby Zion's death. Because of this, when they awarded the Zion estate $750,000 for "Libby Zion's pain and suffering," the jury divided the blame 50/50. This meant they believed Libby was 50 percent culpable for her own death. It also meant the damages against the doctors were reduced by half, to $375,000.

As each verdict was read off, Sidney Zion sat in stunned silence, looking dismayed and then aghast as the foreperson exonerated Ray Sherman for not coming to the hospital that night, and decided in favor of his longtime nemeses on item after item. Halfway through the verdicts, Zion slumped down in his seat and lowered his head onto his chest, raising it to nod in agreement on the few counts he won.

Later, Judge Elliott Wilk threw out Libby Zion's culpability about the cocaine on a technicality and reduced the final damage award against the doctors from $750,000 to $375,000. He did not rule on a Zion motion to dismiss the cocaine verdict for lack of evidence, but approved Zion's motion for a new trial, in which the judge said the Zion side could revisit this issue.

Judge Wilk granted Sidney Zion thirty days to file another motion.

■

During my meeting with Sidney Zion after the verdict, a month or so after he let the retrial deadline pass, the man who now stood at the bar at Gallagher's was much more subdued than the last time we met here. At one point, a flicker of the old fire emerged when he again called New York Hospital "a charnel house." He also said he was shocked by the jury's verdict. "It was a Contract for America jury," he said. "Who would have believed they would say it was okay for Ray Sherman not to show up?" But the passion and Olympian righteousness had mostly disappeared from his voice. It struck me that he looked older—and more sad than angry.

Zion said he was gratified that the judge threw out the cocaine culpability, even if it was on a technicality, though he would have been happier if the judge had ruled in his favor on what he claimed was insufficient evidence. He was also unhappy that the monetary award was smaller than he and many others had expected, saying the $375,000 had been spent long ago on legal fees.*

"What can I say? I wish it had been more clear-cut," he said, shrugging, and sucking deeply on his cigar. "People say we technically won, because we got money out of them. I guess we did." He said, however, that he thought the jury had missed the point about the residency issues, and wondered "how many kids like Libby will die because of this verdict, because we didn't finally put a stop to this insanity."

Given this point of view, I asked him to offer a broader perspective on what he thought was learned from this case.

"What I hope we learned," he said pensively, "is that there are no good hospitals, and maybe there aren't any really bad hospitals; there are careful doctors and negligent doctors. And that's the system. But the system does not account for the difference. The system assumes that they are careful, and nothing protects us from those who are not. We are at the mercy of people who tell us 'We can't do anything about it,' if they tell us anything at all. Mostly, they tell us nothing."

I asked if his crusade to vindicate Libby's death was truly over.

"Yes, it's over," he said with a sigh. "I don't want to go back."

Had the crusade of the last ten years left him weary?

"In fact it saved me. It never took a toll on me," he insisted. "People think it did, but it didn't. What took a toll on me was when they threw in the coke and I knew what a lie it was. But the case itself was a way of motivating me on these residency issues."

Later, though, he admitted that it had been hard to constantly revisit the details of Libby's death. "I say it didn't bother me," he said, "but in one sense it did, because I always had to relive that

---

*After the money was awarded, Zion was able to keep an undisclosed portion, according to his lawyer, Tom Moore.

night. I don't sleep well even now. It never stops. I wake up yelling and screaming sometimes. You don't get over it."

As I left Sidney Zion at Gallagher's on that sticky New York afternoon, smoking his cigar in a corner beneath snapshots of patrons long dead, I wondered if after all these years, Sidney Zion is really willing at last to let his daughter rest in peace.

■

The morning Libby Zion died, a young intern at New York Hospital was almost twenty-four hours into her final thirty-six-hour-shift after a month on the wards. At 7:30, following an exhaustive effort to revive a patient whose heart had stopped, this twenty-seven-yeal-old doctor faced the nightmare of every intern and every physician—a patient had died who probably shouldn't have, a teenager with curly red hair and plump cheeks who a few hours earlier seemed barely sick enough to be in the hospital at all.

The intern, Luise Weinstein, is now thirty-eight years old. She is an associate professor of medicine at Cornell University Medical College and a primary care specialist at New York Hospital. Almost a decade after finishing her residency, Weinstein is seeing patients, attending on the wards, and working to design the hospital's new ambulatory care rotations for residents—all this despite Sidney Zion's best efforts.

Moreover, Weinstein is working in a leading-edge field, ambulatory care, at one of the nation's top hospitals. According to Joseph Hayes, vice chairman of medicine and director of house staff education at The New York Hospital/Cornell, who works closely with Weinstein, she is popular with residents, a good doctor, and a hard worker. "She has gotten a house staff teaching award," he said. "She is absolutely awesome. She's got a walking knowledge of medicine that is unbelievable." Others have found her quiet and very private, with a singleminded devotion to her work. On the witness stand, Luise Weinstein seemed frail; a small, dark-haired woman ready to shrink whenever she was spoken to, though she proved firm and even combative when Zion's lawyer tried to rile her with bombastic, accusatory questions.

But Luise Weinstein is far more than this in the public imagination. For years, she has been the perpetual intern; the forever resident who, until Sidney Zion let his appeal option run out last year, seemed always destined to be the greenhorn who presided when Libby Zion died. To critics of the residency system, she embodied the plight of the resident: tired, stressed, overworked, and unsupervised.

To supporters such as Joseph Hayes, Weinstein was the maligned intern, the innocent victim of medicine's faultfinders and enemies; a talented, even brilliant young doctor wrongly accused. Some of these champions came to this conclusion because they felt it was wrong to blame Weinstein, a mere intern, for systemic problems much bigger than what happened on Payson five during those seven hours in 1984. Others contend that she and the other doctors did nothing wrong that night, period.

Over the course of ten years, Weinstein and the other residents caring for Libby Zion were cleared not only of criminal charges by the grand jury in 1985, but also of charges of professional misconduct by the State Board for Professional Medical Conduct in 1989. State health commissioner David Axelrod, however, added in his letter approving the misconduct board's acquittal that he remained "concerned about the institution's response to the situation leading to Patient A's [Libby Zion's] death with regard to the supervision of interns and residents," and "the division of authority between house staff and others."

When the jury found against her on three counts in the civil trial in 1995, Weinstein stayed quiet and impenetrable in the courtroom. Afterward, she left quickly, making no statements.

■

Luise Weinstein did not lose a daughter on that long ago morning in March. But she did lose a patient, possibly because of administering a drug, Demerol, she has admitted she would not give again to a patient taking Nardil. She denies the Demoral killed Libby, however. In repeated testimony she has steadfastly denied making any other errors, insisting she did nothing wrong when she didn't visit Libby between 3:30 and 6:40 that morning, and didn't call in a supervisor, and didn't order cold compresses to be applied to Libby until shortly before the code. In twelve years, she has never made a public statement about her own feelings concerning the case.

What *did* she feel that morning as she heard the code announced over the intercom on Payson three, walked up the two flights of stairs to Libby's room, worked with the other doctors for fifty minutes in a desperate attempt to revive her, and was unsuccessful? In those moments before the long years of the case began, when she was still simply Dr. Weinstein, one of thousands of anonymous interns then training on America's wards, what was she thinking as she wrote Libby's "Death Note" later that morning in her neat, precise cursive lettering?

Death Note
Patient was found unresponsive, without palpable pulse or spontaneous respiration. Full resuscitation measures were taken, which included intubation, CPR, intravenous pressors, defibrillation . . . despite intubation and oxygenation with 100% O_2, arterial blood gases revealed profound hypoxemia. The patient was pronounced at 7:30 A.M. The attending physician, Dr. Sherman, was notified and will attempt to contact the family. The medical examiner's office was notified.

L. Weinstein

According to the nurses on Payson five, they cried when Libby died. No one saw Luise Weinstein cry; but neither did anyone see Jim Stern shed a tear when Mary Allen suffered as she died. Did Luise Weinstein grieve? Did she step into a supply room, like Stern, and perhaps secretly weep for her patient?

Zion and his lawyer have sometimes depicted Luise Weinstein as a coldhearted, arrogant physician far more interested in writing a correct note than in caring for her patient that night. Zion has repeatedly accused her and the other residents of "killing my daughter." Thomas Moore, Zion's attorney and one of the most successful (and theatrical) malpractice lawyers in the United States today, repeatedly called her in court "an unlicensed, unsupervised first-year postgraduate student," rounding out these words in a booming tenor; a ringing indictment of Weinstein, physicians, and residency programs everywhere.

This seems like a great burden to put on the shoulders of a young woman barely out of medical school, even if she was guilty of lapses that night. Just three days later, Luise Weinstein tested for the final portion of the three-part National Medical Board examination all physicians must pass before being licensed in the United States. This third part specifically examines an intern's practical, clinical knowledge. She scored an amazing 680 on a test where the passing grade is 290, putting her in the ninety-sixth percentile among those taking the exam. Yet as Bertrand Bell has pointed out, Weinstein, Stone, and Maurice Leonard, the R2 in the E.R. who admitted Libby, were virtual novices at the time. He believes they should never have been party to the malpractice suit, insisting that Weinstein was the product of a system that failed her as much as it did Libby Zion.

In discussing the case, Bell talks about the issue of supervision, and the fact that residents are given too much responsibility before they can handle it. He also reiterates his criticism of a system that "kicks out the c.s. factor—the common sense factor.

"If my mother, or you, had seen somebody with a temperature of 103 going up to 104, 105," he told me, "what would you do? You would cool the person down! And she didn't see that because there was no diagnosis and they are taught to never treat symptoms unless you have a diagnosis. She didn't know what she needed to know. But it's not her fault. That is the system."

Sidney Zion asked Bell to testify at the trial, but Bell declined, saying he thought it was wrong for Zion to include the former residents in the suit. "They were kids," said Bell, "neophytes who didn't know any better. What's the point of blaming them?" In a reflective moment, even Zion concedes that Libby's death "is not even all their fault."

■

Taking the stand early in the civil trial, in mid-November 1994, the five-foot-two Weinstein seemed to be weary to the bone of the entire Zion affair, her shoulder-length black hair falling into and nearly obscuring a round, pale face. Dressed in dark, conservative suits and silver earrings, she answered questions during three days on the stand in an almost inaudible, emotionless monotone—except when she became incensed at some of Tom Moore's accusations, and questions she considered annoying. Most of the time, Weinstein spoke without much feeling, glancing off to one side as she repeated information. One of the few times she showed emotion, other than flashing an occasional glare at Tom Moore, was when she talked about the last time she saw

Libby alive. This was during her final day of testimony, when her own lawyer, Frank Bensel, was gingerly walking her through her defense.

Looking toward Bensel, and raising her hand to add emphasis, Weinstein said in a voice raised slightly above her usual whisper: "I spent a lot of time talking to the patient. I was the last person to see and evaluate the patient." Saying that she had given Libby Haldol, a sedative, to calm her, and didn't believe any other treatment was necessary, Weinstein added, looking down and then away from Bensel: "I had hoped . . . that just in a quiet environment, her agitation would cease. We had turned down the lights."

At that moment, Weinstein's inscrutability and her brief, almost monotone style of answering questions seemed to dissolve just a bit.

In a sense, whether or not Luise Weinstein grieved brings us back to Dostoyevsky's question, posed at the beginning of this book: whether it is justifiable to allow a single "tiny creature" to suffer for a greater aim—in this case, so that Weinstein, the never-ending intern, and every other resident could learn something from the death of Libby Zion.

As Sidney Zion says, nothing that has happened since Libby's death—not the grand jury report, the Bell Commission, and what he calls the "Libby Zion Rules"—was worth the death of his daughter. Given that she did die, however, it seems critically important to us all that Luise Weinstein *did* grieve on that chilly morning in March; that before she became the ultimate intern, and her life was changed forever, she paused for a moment to understand the depths of the tragedy that had just happened. Most interns would have been devastated to lose a young, seemingly healthy patient like Libby Zion. I suspect this was the case for Weinstein. Certainly, one hopes—and assumes—she did not simply write her "death note," sign it, and move on to her next task without pondering at least for a moment the bitter reality of what can go wrong, and the sad poetry of what might have been.

■

How important was Sidney Zion's quest?

Zion himself, and most reformers, consider the case a major catalyst for change in New York, and an important vehicle for bringing residency issues to the public's attention. Others dismiss the case as simply the public fumings of a grieving father, with some contending it was at least in part a publicity stunt.

"We learned nothing about house staff education," says The New York Hospital's Joseph Hayes, who insists the reforms of the last ten years would have occurred without the Zion case. He also says that neither hours nor supervision were at issue that night; that Weinstein was not too tired, and was adequately supervised. "I don't know that the supervision that is in place today is any different than it was then. I think we probably now have the attendings spend more time with the house staff than they did," he adds, pointing out that teaching attendings* now spend every morning with interns, rounding and working out daily management issues with each patient. But this new system would not have mattered in the case of Libby Zion, since attendings still are not typically present on the floors at night to directly supervise residents at all times—particularly on a Sunday night, which is when Libby Zion arrived at the E.R. In other words, Hayes seems to be indicating that if another Libby Zion were to appear on Payson five today, she would face a situation similar to what existed the night of March 4–5, 1984: a lone intern supervised by an R2 who might be asleep or on beeper call at home, and an attending, like Sherman, available minutes away, but also asleep or at home and dependent on a resident knowing when to call and what to say.

One huge difference Hayes did not mention is that Libby Zion would almost certainly be seen today by an experienced senior physician at least in the emergency room, where attendings are required to manage cases actively in all New York hospitals twenty-four hours a day. Hayes insists that conditions on the floor, however, have changed but little—and that this is the way it should be, given his belief that Libby Zion did not die from errors committed by the hospital or residents.

But it would be unfair to imply that Joseph Hayes, a lanky, square-jawed physician with an Abe Lincoln beard and a passion for teaching, is a hard-liner blindly defending the old days. His medicine residency program at New York Hospital is among the more progressive I'm aware of.

For starters, he says his program meticulously follows the Bell Rules.

*Hayes's program at The New York Hospital assigns both a teaching attending (or two) and an attending of record for each intern team.

"We don't mess around with the law," claims Hayes, knowing that the hospital where Libby Zion died will always be under closer scrutiny than most. "It's not worth it." According to Hayes, he asks interns on an every-fourth-night call schedule to work twenty-four-hour shifts, with PGY2 or PGY3 night floats taking all admissions after 10 P.M. This allows interns to sleep three or four hours. "This is usually enough," he says, "so that when they make rounds in the morning they are not falling asleep," which he says used to happen. He then gives his postcall residents the day off after morning rounds. "We do not let them go to clinics in the afternoon," says Hayes. "They're tired and their spirits are low. I think it has improved morale."

Hayes also has instituted his own system for formally handing off patients, to facilitate continuity of care. "People would kill for this idea," he says with a grin, letting me peek at a specially designed computer program detailing the status of every patient—which all residents are required to update accordingly, and which they have instant access to from any computer terminal in the hospital. He also has beefed up supervision and didactic teaching by organizing a volunteer corps of attendings to conduct working rounds with interns every morning—that is, to accompany and instruct them while they are checking patients, placing orders, and making decisions. Fellows or attendings are always in-house, he says. Yet the core system at the patient level remains essentially the same as it was in 1984, with an intern in the lead, backed up by an R2—and, since 1993, an R3.

Hayes says these changes would have occurred without the Zion case, and that the timing was coincidental. He also sticks by his belief that, if anything, the case and recent lawsuit "had a negative impact" on residencies.

The *New York Times,* for one, disagrees. In their editorial appearing after the 1995 verdict, the *Times* notes that Sidney and Elsa Zion had "turned their grief into a crusade" and that "A clear public health benefit has flowed from their effort.

"New York became the first state to regulate and limit those notoriously long hours worked by hospital interns and residents," continues the *Times.* "Routine shifts of 36 straight hours were reduced to 24 and work weeks of 100 hours and up were cut to 80. If the verdict [in the civil trial] should now lead to relaxation of state oversight or hospital monitoring of working conditions, the medical profession and the public would suffer.

"The Zions failed to reach their ultimate goal, a large award of punitive damages to make an example of New York Hospital. . . . Still, society now deems these hospital practices unwise and dangerous. The Zion case has educated the public and transformed the working conditions of many hospitals, to the advancement of public safety."

■

The Zion case should not be viewed as an isolated occurrence, however, either in terms of litigation involving residents or attempts at reforming the system. No one knows exactly how many similar lawsuits have been filed, settled, and tried concerning alleged negligence by residents. Again, little data is collected. One study identified ninety-five major suits with a jury verdict between 1975 and 1989, with the verdicts split almost evenly between the resident and the plaintiff. This probably represents only a tiny fraction of the malpractice cases where residents are listed as defendants or codefendants, among the approximately 25,000 to 30,000 malpractice cases filed each year in the United States. None of these cases, however, have had nearly the impact or public involvement as the Zion case—though occasionally there are local suits where the role of a resident becomes a public issue.

Otherwise, calls for reform over the years have come mostly from residents themselves. The first official resident complaint about long hours that I know of occurred while Osler was still alive and teaching at Oxford University in England, where he went after leaving Johns Hopkins in 1905. The year was 1917; the intern was the first female physician ever trained at Bellevue Hospital in New York City, Dr. Connie Guion. After spending a month on back-to-back twenty-four-hour shifts following the hospital's ambulance as its EMT, Guion felt rundown. "She requested of the directors of the hospital that they decrease the number of hours demanded at one time," writes medical historian Carol Lopate in *Women in Medicine*, a request the hospital promptly granted, reducing shifts to just twelve hours.

Guion's initiative was the exception, however, for a system in which interns received no pay, often performed custodial work, handled most of the lab work on the wards, and were expected to be available twenty-four hours a day, seven days a week. Marriage and, in some programs, dating were banned. The word *residents* originates from the fact that trainees literally lived in the hospital. Few complained, since residencies in those days lasted only a year, and virtually all trainees were young white men who thought of their internship as being like a stint in the army: several months of exhausting, scut-filled days spent on the front lines of medicine learning a skill alongside a group of likeminded men, with whom they typically developed strong bonds.

Seventeen years after Dr. Guion's protest, at the height of the Great Depression in 1934, residents launched the first organized efforts at reform. By then, the number of residents in the United States had reached almost 5,000, and the one-year internship was giving way to two years of training, though little else had changed since Guion's day.

"Dissatisfied with no salaries, lack of teaching rounds, and often dangerous working conditions such as ambulance riding," writes medical historian and physician Robert Harmon, "66 intern representatives (known then as internes) from 26 hospitals met in April, 1934, and formed the Interne Council of Greater New York." Two years later, the group went national, opening chapters in Chicago, Boston, Baltimore, and New Jersey, and calling itself the Interne Council of America (ICA). Membership numbered in the hundreds, though by 1940 the ICA was publishing a newsletter with a circulation of some 7,000. During the thirties and forties, the ICA and its successor group, the Association of Internes and Medical Students (AIMS), managed to win modest victories lobbying individual hospitals and states for higher pay ($15 a month in New York in 1935; $60 a month in the United States in 1948), better hospital libraries, and workmen's compensation for interns.*

Then came a period of retrenchment in the late forties and fifties, with the AMA conducting a virulent campaign against AIMS, at one point attacking it as communist during the hysteria then sweeping the country. Claiming the residency group "advocates the overthrow of the United States government by force and violence," staunch conservatives in the AMA accused AIMS of favoring "strikes upsetting to proper medical education," as well as having

---

*During the forties, AIMS leaders included such future luminaries as Arthur Sackler, Leslie Falk, Karl Menninger, and Milton Roemer.

"Communist tendencies," and "Communist affiliations." AIMS denied the charges but lost in droves members who did not want to be associated with an alleged "red" organization. It folded in 1952.

For the remainder of the fifties, virtually all reform talk stopped as medicine rode that decade's extraordinary wave of technological advances, and as academic hospitals exploded in size, with steep increases in beds, research labs, and numbers of residents and faculty. Physician prestige during this period rose to heady heights, and with it a willingness to endure the ordeal of residency to be anointed a member of this temporarily elevated profession. Pragmatically, there was also a tremendous increase in residents going on to specialty fellowships and faculty appointments, which meant one challenged the status quo at the peril of one's career.

Even so, in 1958 the Committee of Interns and Residents, the first true residents' union in the United States, formed in New York City. This was followed over the next five years by unions in Los Angeles and Boston. With the advent of the sixties came another round of activism in what has become a cycle of attempts at reform, small gains, and then lulls. Indeed, after 1965, students in medical schools became as radicalized as their peers on other U.S. campuses, with students and residents campaigning for civil rights, an end to the Vietnam War, and community health projects. Steve Bergman (a.k.a. Samuel Shem) started medical school the summer Richard Nixon admitted to bombing Cambodia, and four students were shot dead by National Guard troops at Kent State. With universities across America striking in protest, Bergman says he and other medical students anguished over whether to join them. "We were just starting to learn the kidney block* when this passionate debate ensued," he remembered. "Half of us saying we can't go out on strike, we'll never learn the kidney. Half of us saying to hell with the kidney, let's go out on strike."

The climate of protest naturally spilled over to residency issues, with several groups of trainees holding demonstrations and making demands. In the sixties, a series of "heal-ins" were held, where residents refused to discharge patients—actions that won pay increases of up to 100 percent, achieved in part because Medicare and Medicaid agreed to fund a sizable share of residents' stipends after its creation in 1965.

This ferment culminated on March 17, 1975, when over 1,500

* "Block" here means a series of classes and labs.

out of 3,000 residents at several New York City hospitals staged the first significant physician strike in U.S. history. The main issue was long hours—and what strike organizers termed the danger to patients of fatigued residents. "It takes an awful lot for a doctor to stay away from a hospital," said Dr. Richard Knutson, a resident and the president of the Committee of Interns and Residents, which organized the job action. Speaking four hours into the three-day strike he told of his "frustration and anger" at the hospitals' refusing their demands to reduce hours and improve working conditions. "We're probably doing more damage every day in the hospital by being overly tired than we can do by taking to the streets."

According to newspaper accounts, patient care was not compromised at the twenty-one affected hospitals, though critics branded the strikers unethical for leaving their patients to join the picket lines. Others insisted the younger generation of doctors was soft and lacked commitment—an argument also leveled at the interns who formed the ICA in 1934. This has continued to be a theme whenever reform pops up.

The strike, however, was notable for two reasons: first, because hospitals agreed to write into residents' contracts that they would work a maximum of every third night on call, rather than the traditional every other night; and second, because the strike—and others held in Los Angeles and Chicago—brought residency reform issues public for the first time. The media pounced on the specter of M.D.'s marching in the streets. Newspapers printed banner headlines following the strike's progress, and published the usual features and profiles of the issues, the strike leaders, and residents and attendings who opposed the action.

One surprising development during the New York strike was the vigorous support of the AMA—which, over the previous decade, had considerably softened its views on residency work issues. In the midst of the strikes and turmoil, they even voted to launch their own residency organization, the Resident Physicians Section (RPS). Officially founded in 1976, the RPS was organized like the AMA itself, with its own system of state delegates meeting twice a year in assemblies. Residents were also allocated seats in the main AMA assembly, and a seat on the Board of Trustees. These measures were enacted in part to rejuvenate a flagging interest among young physicians in the AMA, though they also reflected a deeper recognition by the medical establishment that residents needed a forum to air their complaints.

The tumult of the mid-1970s crescendoed in 1978 with the publication of *The House of God*, an instant bestseller. With its scathing satire of the inhumanity of residency training, *The House of God* reinforced the growing suspicion among some observers and doctors that physician training was not what it should be—and, quite possibly, dangerous. By the early 1980s, on the eve of Libby Zion's death, most nonsurgical programs were switching to every-third-night call. Pay had reached a level of bare subsistence, particularly if one was single. More hospitals were making at least minimal efforts to provide decent sleeping facilities, benefits, and meals while on overnight call—though certainly not all. Some had also added a few basic ancillary services.

Little else had changed, however. Indeed, Connie Guion, the Bellevue intern in 1917, would easily have recognized the residency system in place on March 4, 1984, when Libby Zion was admitted to New York Hospital—though she would have been overwhelmed by the new technologies, and the look of the modern hospital. It's also likely that Guion would have found the training more grueling, given the crush of medical knowledge Luise Weinstein needed to master, and the pressures of tending to much sicker patients than those typically on the wards in 1917.

■

For reasons still not entirely understood, the year of the strikes in New York City and elsewhere coincided with a trend that also sent shock waves through the medical community: the beginning of a steep decline in interest in medicine as a career, as measured by the number of applicants to medical schools. After peaking in 1974 at 42,621 applicants, by 1988 only 26,721 people in the United States wanted to be a doctor enough to file an application—trying for 17,108 positions. Equally alarming to internal medicine educators was a dramatic dropoff in medical students opting for their specialty. By the late eighties, well over half the residency positions available in internal medicine went unfilled.

The fear that the best and brightest were shunning medicine, combined with the Zion case and the bruising debate surrounding the Bell Regulations, left many educators in the late eighties and early nineties feeling troubled and perplexed. Worried about the future of the profession itself, between 1988 and 1993 educators wrote a flurry of soul-searching articles and convened conferences to ask themselves what went wrong. "Where do we go from here?" asked a typical headline in the *Bulletin of New York Academic Medicine* in 1991. "Tinkering or Real Reform? The Choice Is Ours," declared another in the *Annals of Internal Medicine.*

Other studies surveyed young doctors and found that many medical students initially interested in internal medicine had changed their minds after spending time on the medicine wards. What influenced them most, they told researchers, was watching interns chronically exhausted and miserable, and treating a patient population composed mostly of the elderly, the terminally ill, and self-abusers of drugs and alcohol. Then came word in 1991 that even some very prominent programs, including Johns Hopkins—almost exactly a century after William Osler launched the modern training system there—had failed to fill all of their medicine slots for incoming interns during the spring "match."

In Hopkins's case, they quickly filled the slots, and since have had no trouble with the match. But the episode left then chief of medicine at Hopkins, John Stobo, feeling unsettled when I spoke with him soon after the results were announced. Sitting in downtown Baltimore in an office dominated by an enormous oil painting of his predecessor, William Osler, Stobo seemed genuinely distressed about the state of medical training across the country.

A small, lean man with a sharp profile, thinning hair, and a disarmingly direct style of speaking, Stobo told me that reforms in his program up until that time had been "fine tuning." Referring in part to the surprise of not filling the match, he said that two years earlier he and other senior educators had considered making changes in the program, but decided not to. "But this year," he said, "it became clear to us that we have to. The mandate is for substantial change, change not for the sake of change."

Reforms Stobo was considering included more didactic training, more time in the clinics with outpatients, practical training in preventive medicine and how to handle patients' social problems, a reduced patient load, and additional backup staff. He also wanted to involve medical schools in his reforms, insisting that "more and more students come into residency training ill prepared" for the practicalities of being a doctor.

"The whole system of how we train physicians is archaic," he concluded, "and rapidly becoming a dinosaur."

■

In the midst of this anguish among educators, I attended the June 1991 AMA meeting in Chicago. Held in the cavernous, marble-paneled halls of the Chicago Hilton, the meeting was dominated in part by yet another cyclical upswing in residency activism—the climax of some five years of agitation triggered by the Zion case, and the implementation of the Bell Regulations two years earlier in New York.

For two days, I followed the latest company of would-be resident-reformers bustling about the wide, ornate hallways, busily attending meetings and caucuses. They conferred with AMA leaders, held hasty negotiations in backrooms, attended delegate assembly sessions, and convened two remarkable public seminars. One was titled "Resident Physician Abuse," which turned into a "true confessions" session of residents and even attendings recounting horror stories of trainees elbowed and shoved by attending surgeons, forced to work seventy-two-hour shifts and longer, and kicked out of programs for no good reason—in one case, because a surgical resident had a colleague cover for him while his wife was in advanced labor and suffering potentially life-threatening complications. The other seminar was a debate between New York surgeon Frank Spencer, then president of the American Board of Surgeons, and California resident Rebecca Patchin, the RPS delegate to the AMA's main assembly. The debate remained cordial but gave air to the sizable gulf separating resident activists from traditionalists who believed the system needed little or no reform of hours, supervision, or educational emphasis. As I mentioned earlier, Spencer agreed that residents were overworked, but blamed scut and economics. He insisted that fatigue was not a danger to patients, and that physicians should be always available for their patients, regardless of drowsiness or illness.

Patchin and her group of resident-reformers were far more polite and neatly coiffed than the demonstrators in 1975, who shared that decade's propensity for unruly hair, muttonchops, and rabble-rousing talk. Their leader was RPS chairperson Laurie McKeown, a lean, dark-haired, no-nonsense surgical resident from the Mayo Clinic in Rochester, Minnesota. As I met with her between meetings, she spoke in sound bites, saying things like: "The training of resident physicians has been called the last great sweatshop in America," and "Many of us think that fatigue is a violation of the Hippocratic Oath—Do no harm. We are concerned that a fatigued resident violates this."

McKeown and other residents explained that they had just spent several months painstakingly negotiating with the AMA and the Accreditation Council for Graduate Medical Education (ACGME)— the body that accredits residency programs—haggling over reform language in the two organizations' codes and regulations. She thrust at me an AMA document, "Report KKK," outlining the AMA's policy on residency work hours reform, and where the issue then stood.

"All residents should, on average, be able to have at least one twenty-four-hour day out of seven free of patient care responsibilities," said the report, quoting AMA policy, "and should be on-call in the hospital no more than every third night when averaged over a four-week period."

McKeown called these provisions "minimally acceptable," and "a start," but noted with a sigh that even these very modest reforms—which striking residents in 1975 thought they had won sixteen years earlier—were being vehemently opposed by four specialties, whose Residency Review Committees had the power to accept or to veto proposed changes in the ACGME code governing the accreditation of their own programs. "These are all surgical," said McKeown in a frustrated voice, "the four most abusive. They refuse to even answer our questionnaires."

According to Report KKK, presented by Dr. Joseph Painter, chairman of the AMA's Board of Trustees, the leaders of the surgical specialties had "evidenced knowledge of and concern for work load, moonlighting, inattention to personal needs such as nutrition, sleeping quarters, safety and security, debt, family demands, lack of adequate support systems and other issues." Even so, wrote Painter—trying to sound conciliatory, but unable to mask his own impatience—the surgical specialties "have not adopted the guidelines."

McKeown considered Painter's statement about the surgeons' "concern" as "meaningless" until they accepted these minimal work-hour reforms. "Change is very slow," she said, noting that substantial reform was still a distant goal. "The changes we are asking for now are minor. I'm afraid that real reform will come about after we are dead."

■

Concern for their young colleagues' well-being—and patient safety—were not the only issues driving the AMA's interest in reform that summer. There was also the palpable fear that states other than New York would soon impose Bell-style regulations on a profession bitterly opposed to any and all outside controls. According to Report KKK, since 1988 nine states had considered legislation to regulate residencies, with five still actively pursuing government intervention. These included California, Massachusetts, and Illinois. These three states, along with New York, train over one-third of all residents in the country. Three other states, said KKK, had tabled legislation pending the outcome of the proposed ACGME rules.

"There is significant support for an extreme bill in California," said RPS delegate Brian Greenberg, a (neatly) bearded, soft-spoken but energetic resident in pediatrics at UCLA Medical Center in Los Angeles. "They want to do more than in New York," he added, saying that the bill in Sacramento would not only duplicate the Bell Regulations but would also regulate hours residents sleep, and the content of their workday. Greenberg later said this bill came close to passing at the committee level in 1992 in the California Assembly, and almost passed again the following year.

■

Despite frustrations about the slow pace of change, however, most resident leaders left Chicago believing that at least minimal reforms were on the verge of happening.

And so they did. In 1993, the ACGME added to its mandatory accreditation requirements—with the surgeons' grudging approval —provisions limiting call to no more than every third night, with one day in seven free of hospital duties. They also added requirements about adequate supervision and limiting service that were vague on specifics, but made it clear that programs would face censure if they blatantly ignored supervision and overloaded residents with scut.

In the end, the surgeons were swayed by the prospect of even more onerous rules being imposed by state governments—something that failed to happen outside of New York, as legislators succumbed in other states to AMA and hospital lobbyists' promising to follow the new ACGME rules voluntarily. Lawmakers were also scared off from passing Bell-style rules when they saw the nearly $200 million annual price tag in New York, particularly in a period of deep recession and massive deficits in California and Massachusetts. It also seemed likely that the federal government would incorporate resident issues into the great debate then picking up momentum in 1993 and 1994 as President Bill Clinton proposed to overhaul the entire health care system.

■

Since passage of the ACGME rules in 1992, reform has swung into another lull.

"I suspect that we reached a saturation point with what we could do," explains Brian Greenberg, now a private practice pediatrician in Tarzana, California, and a member of the board of the California Medical Association. "Plus you had people who said, 'Gee, we already made some incremental change. Let's see what happens over the next couple of years.' "

It's now been *more* than a couple of years—and perhaps time to judge the success of the reforms that emerged from the Zion and Bell era. As usual, data is sparse. According to Steve Ellwing, staff director for the AMA's resident physician section, "The hours are a little better, although it depends on where you are." New York's department of health has commissioned a group of researchers from Johns Hopkins and other institutions to survey residents in their state on how well they think the Bell Regulations are working, but the results will not be available for some time.

Meanwhile, in New York we do have the raw data from state investigations into compliance with the Bell Regulations. As I mentioned earlier, these suggest that some programs are not always following the rules on supervision and hours. Moreover, the basic system in New York has not really changed dramatically since 1984, with hours reduced some, and supervision still largely at arm's length at many hospitals, despite the presence of more attendings and fellows at night.

The fate of voluntary guidelines put in place in the early nineties is even more difficult to assess. I know of no studies, period, though there is a gathering body of anecdotal evidence and perceptions from residents, and from officials at the ACGME and AMA, that some programs continue to flaunt even the minimal ACGME rules.

Many programs have introduced reforms, particularly in internal medicine and pediatrics, where an every-fourth-night call is now the norm, and night floats and caps are growing more common. Efforts to beef up ancillary services in some hospitals have helped, too. Yet this hardly means all of the more than 7,200 residency programs in the United States are where they should be, even according to the rules—particularly when it comes to supervision. Indeed, most programs I observed remain stubbornly and fundamentally entrenched in the old plunge-in method despite modest improvements, with residents seldom seeing their attendings on the wards, and senior residents continuing to supervise juniors one or two years below them. Scut also continues to absorb 20 percent or more of a trainee's time, with residents overwhelmed by caseloads that have declined only a little, if at all, since 1991.

According to Brian Greenberg, only a few programs in his state have fully implemented voluntary guidelines drafted by California educators in the early 1990s to head off passage of Bell-style laws. In some cases, Greenberg says, the rules have been ignored. "If the guidelines had been implemented," he adds wistfully, "that would have solved everything."

Judy Linger, a psychiatry resident at the University of Kentucky at Lexington, and the current chairperson of the AMA's resident physician section, says that nationally the voluntary reforms have also been erratic. "We were able to get the wording into the general requirements for the ACGME that specifically outlines what programs can and cannot ask a resident to do," she says. "The problem is that residents are still being asked to do these things [they shouldn't]. We want to start getting programs to enforce the rules. There are still surgical programs that are asking residents to do every-other-night call for months and months at a time, without time off. And you also have the physical challenges of attendings who are verbally abusive or harassing the residents."

According to the ACGME's John Gienapp, violations of supervision provisions rank as a "significant and frequent citation." Duty hours violations are also a "significant citation." He did not have exact figures, but said that at any given time 2 percent to 3 percent

of all residency programs in the United States are on probation—
many of them in part because of hours and supervision violations.
Other programs are cited for hours and supervision violations, but
have retained their accreditation because the ACGME typically
shuts down programs only after repeated patterns of numerous violations.

"We have never shut down a program, that I can recall, for one
thing alone," said Gienapp. "Usually it's several things."

As for abuse, Linger and other resident leaders cite surveys where
up to 90 percent of residents and medical students report being
abused and harrassed by more senior physicians; with 24 to 52 percent saying they received a "threat of physical harm," and 50 percent
of women reporting "unwanted sexual advances." A 1994 report
from the AMA, published in *JAMA*, calls on teaching hospitals and
residency programs to "establish formal mechanisms for handling
complaints of incompetence, impairment, and unethical conduct."

If what Linger and other residency leaders say is true, then resident ire and frustration loom as large as ever. There are rules on the
books, they say, but no way to truly enforce them, or to report programs in violation without endangering one's career.

"We are trying to figure out a way to help residents report those
programs that are still abusing the system," says Linger, "in a way
where there won't be any repercussions for the resident. If a resident is seen as a rabble-rouser or troublemaker," she adds, "they
can make that resident's life pretty miserable."

At Linger's own hospital, she said, the surgery residents "are still
asked to work every-other-night or every-third-night call for
months at a time. And they are in a pyramid system and there is a
tremendous fear to do anything to call attention to yourself that
would be perceived as negative by the department. Each year residents are dropped from the total program because they start with
five entry-level residents, but they only graduate two or three at the
end of a five-year program. When you have that kind of pressure
over your head, you don't complain about the work environment.
You don't complain about how many nights it's been since you have
been able to see your family."

"I get an awful lot of calls from people who are in trouble with their programs," said the AMA's Steve Ellwing. "Some of them because they complained about hours, or supervision, or other program abuses." A few, he said, are in trouble with their programs because they are "bad doctors," or for other "legitimate" reasons. But others have real complaints, he says, and will ask Ellwing advice on whether to file a complaint with either their hospital or the ACGME.

"I frequently advise people that are in trouble in their programs not to file a complaint," says Ellwing, "because you are having enough trouble now trying to survive in the first place. I tell them they're playing a game of cards, and the program director has all of the aces. The residents have only small cards."

Linger points out that there is no real mechanism for residents to file complaints if they are harassed or fired improperly, particularly if their program or hospital is not taking ACGME rules of due process in grievance procedures seriously. For instance, she said it was "normal for the program director, who will be the person kicking the resident out of the program, to be on the panel that hears their grievance." Nor does the ACGME—or anyone else—handle individual complaints. "They will look at a situation from an accreditation point of view," said Ellwing, "and say you didn't get due process. And they'll slap the program on the hand and say we are going to watch them, but that's the most you are going to get out of it. The only other recourse is a lawsuit."

Take the case of a PGY6 in a specialty surgery residency whom I'll call James Dooley. Placed on probation at the end of his fifth year primarily because he did badly on an in-service exam, Dooley passed a makeup exam and was allowed to proceed to his sixth and final year as a chief resident. Just three months into his chief year, however, he was dismissed, with the program contending that he continued to perform poorly.

According to Dooley, his termination occurred after a series of incidents with a prominent attending at one of his program's hospitals, where Dooley was training that summer and fall. Claiming there was a personality conflict with the attending, Dooley charges that this senior surgeon at one point ordered him to leave the O.R. during a procedure. Soon after, Dooley also insists that this attending took him aside early in his rotation, swore at him, and said, "everybody . . . hates you and you really piss off them and me. You are a nasty human being, and I am going to have you fired." Sources at the hospital* say the attending denies having said this, insisting the opposite—that he actually went out of his way to help Dooley overcome his alledged difficulties. My sources also insist that the program tried hard to help Dooley keep up, but that the chief and senior educators were unwilling to drop him back a year or two when they believed he would not be ready to graduate the following summer. Dooley, however, points out that he passed his makeup exam, and contends that he fulfilled all requirements he was aware of during his probation period. He also believes that his low score on the in-service exam was an embarrassment to his program, and that this may have been another reason he was let go.

The James Dooley I spoke with is angry and frustrated about what has happened to him, but he seems a reasonable person—an assessment officials at the AMA and ACGME who have reviewed his case, and spoken with him, agree with. But even if he was truly "a nasty human being"—and if these words were actually spoken—this is not a basis for firing him, though a charge of incompetence is.

Dooley, however, claims that he was considered competent enough to repeatedly be allowed to operate solo, and to supervise more junior residents. Indeed, neither his chief nor any of the senior physicians in his department have ever officially accused him of incompetence, with sources at the hospital assuring me the chief considers Dooley a competent physician. Apparently, not every surgeon in the program agreed with this, though Dooley has had several attendings champion him, contending that he should not have been terminated.

After the firing, the chairman of Dooley's former department claimed a grievance hearing was not required, despite ACGME regulations requiring due process, though the department grudgingly granted Dooley one anyway. The hearing was delayed, however, for seven months while Dooley waited in limbo, unable to continue his training.

After an initial session, and a lawsuit filed by Dooley, the hearing was suspended pending a settlement in which the hospital proposed to pay Dooley's legal fees in exchange for his formally withdrawing

---

*Neither the physicians nor the hospital were able to comment on specifics of this case, citing reasons of confidentiality.

from the program. Meanwhile, Dooley found another position as a resident at a hospital 2,000 miles away, he says with the help of one of his supporters in the department.

During this process, Dooley contacted the ACGME to see if they could help. According to an ACGME official, they sympathize with Dooley. But they can do nothing to help him in his specific allegations, though the official said that the ACGME was planning to look into the due process system at Dooley's former program during its next scheduled investigation.

After the proposed settlement, Dooley thought the matter was over. However, even as he moved to his new city, the chief of his old program sent off a form to the licensing board in Dooley's new state claiming he had reservations about Dr. Dooley's competence to practice medicine and surgery. Apparently, this triggered a competency hearing, delaying the issuance of a state license for Dooley, and jeopardizing his new slot, since the state could not act until several weeks after the residency was scheduled to begin.

Dooley's former chief has insisted that he never intended to cause trouble for this young doctor. When he found out about the hearing and the delay, he sent a letter to the state licensing authorities insisting that Dooley really was competent to be a physician—a letter that might be interpreted as a reversal of his previously stated "reservations." Sources close to the chief deny this, however. Officials at the state board would not comment on what caused the hearing to be called, or the license to be held up. On February 6, 1995, the state issued Dooley's license, though by then he had lost his residency position in the new program. He currently is moonlighting at emergency rooms trying to pay his sizable legal bills, while he awaits word on whether he will be accepted in another residency program in yet another state.

"I'm very upset," says Dooley. "It's my belief that I did not deserve what I got. But I have to keep going, to get my life in order so I can move on."

∎

The perception that reform has failed in many instances has provoked another group of residents to confront the same problem Connie Guion complained about at Bellevue in 1917—and the same issues the ICA lobbied for in 1934, and AIMS in the 1940s, and the strikers in 1975, and Sidney Zion and the Bell Commission in the 1980s—that residents are being overworked, underpaid, and can present a needless danger to patients. "There is a feeling that there still is a problem," said Ellwing, "and that it is time to look at this again." He said the current leaders of the RPS were in the midst of deciding strategy. "What should we do about work hours?" he said. "Do we want to attack it again, and do we look at it from a different perspective perhaps than ACGME?"

∎

Clearly, reform over the years has helped, though the story is as much one of nonreform—and fierce resistance, weak enforcement, a rapid turnover of resident activists, and, in some cases, a denial that reform is required. This is why the issues of hours and all the rest keep coming back, as fresh generations of residents discover to their astonishment a system still not as conducive to learning, patient safety, and their own health as it might be.

As Steve Ellwing put it, "These are old issues that have been addressed before, but that still seem to be on the forefront because residents feel that they have no real control over their own lives." They also "think it is very difficult to remain compassionate; to be involved with their patients. That is a big complaint, that they really want to be caring physicians, but you reach a point where it is tough to care, and expediency takes over."

Perhaps only one thing has truly and unequivocally changed for the better in recent years—that as wave after wave of complaints, anguish, and frustration have struck at an intransigence seemingly as immovable as Mount Everest, *attitudes* have slowly shifted. No longer does the AMA claim resident activists are reds trying to overthrow the government. Nor are residency complaints routinely pushed aside anymore by the AMA, ACGME, and other influential physician groups that have gone on record acknowledging there are problems. Yet many young doctors today are dismayed and frustrated with having to make the same choice faced by Connie Guion in 1917—between their own survival and what's best for their patients.

Another problem stems from the fact that residency is a tempo-

rary condition—and that while residents are training, they have little or no time to think about reform, or much else beside their
immediate duties. Consequently, the sort of long-term, persistent
and time-consuming action necessary for basal change remains elusive. "I think these things would happen if the residents demanded
them," said John Stobo of Hopkins, who said he would like to see
more resident demands for certain reforms. "But I don't hear them
doing this," he said, talking about Hopkins. When I suggested to
him this might be because they were too tired and busy, he said,
"Of course, that may be one reason."

Despite all the talk of reform, little today matches the common-
sense reaction of Bellevue educators in 1917, when they decided a
twenty-four-hour-a-day, seven-day-a-week shift following an ambulance was a bad idea. Indeed, they didn't wait a few decades, conduct dozens of studies, and then decide to voluntarily cut back to,
say, twenty-two hours, hoping this would resolve the issue. Though
no one would want to go back to conditions in 1917, in this
instance educators acted decisively, and cut the hours on this service in half.*

A doctor who spoke to Sidney Zion shortly after the verdict in
his trial has possibly offered the most prescient insight of all. With
Zion in shock over the jury's failure to find against the hospital on
the issues of supervision, fatigue, and inexperience—and on the
matter of cocaine—this physician told him not to be discouraged.

" 'It's a century-long war,' " Zion says the doctor told him, " 'and
you've fired the first shot.' "

Maybe he's right; medicine is progressing, but only very, very
slowly. Which again raises the question I've been asking all along: is
this acceptable? Are there no creative solutions?

---

*Admittedly, one reason for Bellevue's decisiveness was that it cost the hospital nothing, since
additional residents were paid the going wage of the day—nothing.

CHAPTER 10

Common Sense:
A Blueprint for Change

To dare: that is the whole secret of revolutions.

Antoine Saint-Just

Albert Most sits at the pinnacle of a pyramid that has ruled academic medicine since William Osler's day. Chief of medicine at Rhode Island Hospital, fifty-seven-year-old Most trained in the early sixties at Johns Hopkins Medical School, then moved to City Hospital in Boston for his residency and a fellowship in cardiology.

Tall and powerful-looking, with a strong chin and silver hair combed back like that of a leading man still handsome in middle age, Most has directed medicine at this Brown University–affiliated hospital since 1987. In one of the more reformed programs in the country, Al Most in 1990 switched the eighty residents in his department from a classic every-third-night thirty-six-hour shift to a schedule of every fourth night, with night floats and caps.* Residents are also allowed at least one in every seven days off, and often two.

This switch occurred during Jennifer Jeremiah's third year of residency at Rhode Island. (Jeremiah is the attending who cuts her clinical work in half during months she supervises on the wards at Rhode Island.) "The students and residents were very vocal about changing things," remembers Jeremiah, "and they listened, and implemented things right away. This program is known for emphasizing quality of life for the residents, and not letting it sacrifice a good education." Rhode Island's program has no official twenty-four-hour attendings in-house, and some ancillary services affecting residents could be improved. But in terms of work hours and patient load, Al Most's program fully complies (and then some) with the minimal rules required by organized medicine.

For Al Most, however, this is not enough. He wants to try what

*In Rhode Island's intensive care units, shifts are twenty-four hours on and twenty-four hours off.

amounts to a revolutionary change, something he calls a "no night-call system." He insists this is a logical reaction to a pattern of incremental reform, which has doggedly attempted to preserve the old notion of a trainee always fielding whatever patients came through the door—a forever on-duty novitiate essentially "residing" in the hospital. This system, Most contends, is straining mightily as programs stretch out the time between call nights and then try to cram in a crush of admissions all in one long, grueling call "day" of up to thirty-six hours. In other words, three or four days of admissions are now compressed into one.

"At this hospital," says Most, "we've already done all the things you might reasonably do to make the workplace manageable. But the more you stretch out the number of nights on, the more you have to do on that night on call to deliver enough work so that it adds up to a sufficient quantum of patients." He says his residents often have to work up five new patients or more in a single call night. "I think that's too many," he contends, recalling that when he was a resident, working up five patients in a single call night was "heroic beyond belief."

"The way I would envision it," explains Most, "you have eight interns, and they would be taking patients in turn, and you could calculate out how many they should get each day—ten, say. Eight residents get ten admissions. And if they all got their patients by eight o'clock, and got their work done, they could all go home." Night floats would take over in the evening, as they do now, he says. And interns could stay late if they needed to, or to follow through on a clear issue of continuity of care. "If they stay late," he says, "some people might want to sleep here, rather than drive home late. But usually, they would be home."

I suggested to Most that many of his fellow chiefs would find the "no call" idea unacceptable. "I know of chiefs who consider night floats radical," I said. "Now you're talking about turning the residency into essentially a day job." I asked Most how to convince traditionalists that the "no-call" is not further diluting the commitment to always be there for your patient.

"In the purest sense," Most said, leaning in and obviously relishing this argument, "you stay with your patient—but how long? twelve hours? twenty-four hours? forty-eight hours? There's a point when people go home. They have families, they eat, life goes on. You're a doctor, not a sprinkler system that's always got to be operational. There is a limit. Staying that first night with your patient is very traditional. It's a belief with no proven merit to it. I understand it. I remember staying up all night, but even staying up until two at night, and then having to get up for work the next day, you get very tired. This was not a good thing. I didn't like it, I couldn't perform at my best."

■

Sitting in his office, under shelves packed with journals, Most's large frame barely fits on a small couch. He leans forward when he talks, emphasizing points with his hands. He is an excellent listener, too, sitting back with the slow grace of an old-style gentleman—polite, encouraging, his face moving from smiles to seriousness to concern in a way that reminded me of something that Tom Delbanco once told me. He said that physicians need to become chameleons with their patients, responding empathetically to their emotions, hopes, and fears of the moment. I suppose this also holds true for pedagogues.

Al Most's mannerisms seem to mirror his philosophy of medicine: that there must be one part aggressiveness and forthrightness, and one part empathy; with a willingness to listen and to allow input, whether it comes from a resident, attending, or patient. This suggests another element to Most's proposed "revolution": a teaching and management style that Bertrand Bell refers to as the "c.s. factor," and what philosophers for centuries have called "moderation in all things" and "the virtue of the mean."

Aristotle—a physician's son—dubbed it "The Golden Mean." Writing soon after Hippocrates' death some 2,300 years ago, Aristotle wrote: "A mean is that which is defined by a rational principle, such as a man of practical wisdom would use to determine it. It is the mean by reference to two vices: the one of excess and the other of deficiency." Following the mean, he adds, "makes a man good, and makes him do his work well."

This sums up in essence the arguments posed by Bell, Delbanco, Most—and to a certain extent by Osler and Flexner—that excess is bad, senseless, and even dangerous, particularly when defended by traditionalists who insist it represents the only way.

At Rhode Island, I saw the "c.s. factor" at work when Jennifer Jeremiah attended on the wards—teaching, listening, and combining understanding with forcefulness, such as when she compelled an intern to present a patient by memory because she knew this PGY1 was ready and needed to learn the discipline of truly knowing her patients.

"That intern is going to be tougher," says Most, when I tell him what Jeremiah did, "and I mean that in a good sense. That person will be better able to deal with challenges because she has been pushed a little bit. Because she can do it. She can do the presentation without the notes." This is what the art of teaching is all about, according to Most and the others: to know when to push, to shape a trainee to evolve in his or her knowledge and skills.

The end product of Most's and Jeremiah's style of education is someone like Peg Miller, a PGY1 when I met her, who has just finished her residency at Rhode Island. A gentle woman with large brown eyes and an enviable steadiness, Peg insisted on spending more time with patients and their families than most of the residents I followed. But she could also be tough; she demanded a surgical intern remove a drainage tube inserted into an HIV-positive patient's chest longer than she thought was necessary, especially for a man whose immune system might not be able to fight off an opportunistic infection. It was Peg hounding the surgical resident that finally got the tube removed.

Perhaps even more important, in Most's wards, clinics, and ICUs I frequently heard residents admitting what they didn't know—asking questions and posing solutions in an environment where they weren't made to feel like idiots because they didn't yet know how to insert a central line, work up a fever, or operate a ventilator.

"Having residents in the hospital is always a risk," observes Al Most. "They should never be in a position to do harm. We have layers of supervision, but it only works if a resident knows when he doesn't know. When I was a resident, there was an ironman mentality about calling for help. That's ridiculous. You call for help if you need it. I think we do a good job here of making the residents feel they can do this."

■

Most is not alone in talking about significant reform, though he seems to be going farther than most educators I'm aware of in trying to implement his ideas. Last spring, he ran an experiment, shifting one of his ward teams to a no night-call system. "It didn't work as well as I hoped," he said, "in part because the chief residents made the schedule too complex." Some of the residents also resisted the change, he said, unhappy because they missed having the "good" days under the old system—days with no call.

"Residents are sometimes the most conservative people around," said Most, recalling that there was stiff opposition among some of the house staff in 1990, when he switched to a night float. "They learn what it takes to make it through the system, and don't like it when the rules change. But try taking away the night float today. There would be riots. They love it."

He maintains that he hasn't given up on his no night-call and other ideas. "From an educational standpoint, it's still where I want to be," said Most. "It also should make life much easier for the residents. Next time, we'll work a little harder to include everyone in advance, and to simplify things." Meanwhile, Most's program may remain less than his ideal, but at least he is genuinely attempting to bridge the gulf between stated principles and everyday practice.

■

Other programs remain stalled in the talk stage. For instance, Johns Hopkins's medicine department has yet to implement many of John Stobo's plans. In part, this is because Stobo relinquished his position as chief of medicine to become the chairman and CEO of Johns Hopkins Healthcare, an alliance of Baltimore hospitals joining forces to draw in managed care contracts. He is also vice dean for clinical sciences. "On a scale of one to ten," he noted, "I got to about three-and-a-half in what I wanted to change in the medicine department."

Stobo is perhaps being too hard on himself. During his tenure, he did switch to an every-fourth-night call from every third, increased ancillary backup and nurse clerks to assist residents, and improved on-call rooms. He also introduced more ambulatory care rotations—though not nearly enough, he says. Still, the core of his former program remains unchanged since we first spoke in 1991, with thirty-six-hour shifts, and, he says, no caps or night floats.

Hopkins is not alone. In Jim Stern's program, residents continue to take call every third night on some rotations, but now have a night float to take admissions after midnight. Rotations through the ICUs have also been reduced slightly, with more time added to ambulatory shifts.

Stobo concedes that the reforms at Hopkins and elsewhere are hardly earth-shattering. Indeed, at some institutions even incremental and obvious solutions to the work-hours issue continue to be regarded as radical and unproved. For instance, I know educators who still consider night floats overly experimental, fearing they will interfere adversely with continuity of care. Yet night floats have been around at least since the 1940s, when Bob Nye trained at Rochester's Strong Memorial Hospital—one of the finest teaching hospitals in the country—and was able to sleep at night because his service had a night float. At Boston City, Al Most says he also trained under a night float system back in the sixties. Indeed, numerous studies detailing night-float strategies suggest that having a team on late at night to take admissions and cover patients can be successful.

For example, a study in *Academic Medicine*, by onetime Surgeon General nominee Henry W. Foster, M.D., and his colleague Vicki L. Seltzer, M.D., concluded after surveying OB–GYN programs across the country that (1) creative scheduling was possible; and (2) "A key feature necessary to implement the new type of schedule is the use of a night float system." Foster and Seltzer suggest that night floats used properly could reduce the workweek for obstetrics residents to about seventy hours a week, without impacting training or patient care.

Other studies, from Vanderbilt University to the University of Oklahoma, and Tufts University to the University of North Carolina, suggest that fewer hours, innovative scheduling, better supervision, and other workplace reforms such as maternity leave and sick-day coverage, have improved resident morale and not adversely impacted patient care or education.

A few educators have also tried to significantly reshape their curriculum—to increase supervision and direct teaching; to better balance outpatient and inpatient rotations; and to add more meaningful clinical ethics and humanities components. Some have suggested that medicine return to a one-year or two-year residency for a general primary care physician. Others have proposed going back to the very beginning of a physician's training in medical school, and linking the book training phase more intimately with hands-on clinical teaching—in other words, eliminating the current barrier between the student and resident phases. This would hclp alleviate a complaint I frequently hear from residency directors and chief of services: that even after four years of medical school, many arriving interns know so little practical medicine, they cannot take a patient history, read a simple X ray, or tap on an abdomen to check a patient's liver. This is one reason why Bertrand Bell has proposed putting off the awarding of an M.D. until the end of residency and a successful completion of qualifying exams. "Often these people are not really doctors," Bell wrote of residents in a 1995 *New York Times* editorial, "at least in the sense that the public understands: experienced, board-certified physicians and surgeons. They are graduate medical students."

Medical schools from Harvard to the University of Pittsburgh have experimented over the past half decade on integrating the wards and clinics with the classroom and lab, with mixed results. Many medical schools today insert even first-year students into a clinical setting. Others, like Harvard Medical School, have tried teaching "modules," integrating textbooks, labs, and real patients, though apparently a backlash is gathering among some Harvard educators who believe this is diluting basic science instruction, which traditionally has dominated the first two years of medical school. Many other programs remain unconvinced.

Even the vaunted new emphasis on ambulatory care is so far an embryonic revolution. According to the most recent *Directory of Family Practice Residency Programs*, virtually every program listed is still heavily weighted toward inpatient care, with most programs offering only about 20 percent of their rotations to clinics and other outpatient settings—this in programs *specializing* in primary care. This is despite calls since at least 1992 to increase outpatient training time to 50 percent of a primary care resident's year. Educators such as Al Most, Joseph Hayes, and John Stobo point out that outpatient content is steadily increasing, though many academic hospitals are facing financial barriers to expanding their outpatient base. Either they lack the funds to build more clinics, or they have been unable to compete with nonteaching hospitals and clinics to draw in the healthy, insured patients vital to a hospital's bottom line in this new age of managed care.

Another problem has been pointed up by an attending who manages an outpatient clinic in Seattle. He told me that one of the great frustrations of training in urban areas, where most teaching hospitals are located, is the high prevalence of patients who are drug and alcohol abusers, smokers, and have other self-destructive pathologies. "Even in clinics, you are getting a preponderance of this group," he said. "You also get a high no-show rate for abusers who just don't come in. This means you may have ten patients scheduled, and only three show up. This is bad training, and very frustrating, because these problems are caused by socioeconomic factors beyond the reach of a concerned resident."

One wonders how this will affect the much talked about statistic that for the first time in decades, in 1995, 27.6 percent of medical school seniors wanted to go into primary care.* This is good news, given that just three years ago, the number was only 14.6 percent. Another hopeful sign is a small but expanding movement to send residents into satellite clinics, private physicians' offices, and other outpatient sites far away from downtown wards and clinics, where they work with senior physicians and patients in settings much closer to what most will operate in after finishing their training. Programs are also increasing month-long blocks of time devoted exclusively to outpatient care.

Yet this new, hopeful cohort of potential primary care doctors must still survive an educational experience topheavy with technology, specialties, and inpatient care—and an outpatient experience that may be less appealing than they expect. New residents will also be as susceptible as always to the seductions of high-tech medicine that has lured away many professed generalists in the past, though one of the advantages of managed care is that primary care doctors are no longer looked down on by some of their specialist colleagues. Indeed, in 1994, primary care was one of the few "specialties" where salary growth did not decline.

Still, a study just last fall in *Pediatrics* cites data suggesting an overwhelmingly lukewarm response to implementing serious outpatient programs (called "continuity clinics," or "CCs"). "Many residency programs," conclude the authors, "have not provided the required priority, protected time, or adequate resources for CCs." Indeed, as long as a resident's "real work" is perceived to be on the wards—where he or she is, after all, the primary doctor for demand-

*The current ratio of primary care physicians to specialists in the United States is about 20:80.

ing, very sick patients—afternoons or a day or two a week relegated to a hospital outpatient clinic will do nothing to squelch the attitude of "Why am I checking for hay fever in this patient when I've got twelve people on the ward who could crash at any time?" One resident I spent time with in a clinic called this the "Let me do my real work" mentality.

■

In the summer of 1994, I visited St. Thomas's Hospital in London, across the Thames from Parliament and Big Ben. In our discussions over tea and cake, Dr. Colin Stern, dean of postgraduate education, did *not* talk about possible reforms. He explained what reforms were already in place in Britain—including a seventy-two-hour workweek being gradually winnowed down to fifty-six hours, and greatly increased how-to didactic sessions with specially assigned physician-tutors, whose primary job is to teach. "The emphasis here is more on individual teaching than in America," said Stern, who bristled at the idea that Britain might be teaching substandard physicians by cutting down to seventy-two or fifty-six hours. "We are known at St. Thomas for producing excellent doctors," he said, explaining that Parliament and the public have demanded residents work fewer hours—and, perhaps as important, the British government has provided the funding to make it happen.

Britain is not alone among Western nations initiating real reforms, including limits on resident work hours. For instance, all European Union countries are presently required to restrict workloads in the hospital to seventy-two hours. Ontario in Canada has a limit of sixty hours; in Denmark and other Scandinavian countries, residents officially work only thirty-seven hours a week; in New Zealand, the numbers are forty hours for nonward rotations and fifty hours when students are on the wards.

Problems exist with reform in these systems. For instance, medical educators in Britain told me that house officers in some hospitals are still expected to work overtime. A junior attending in London said they are "often required to volunteer," but at least they are paid market wages for overtime far higher than their usual hourly stipend. The same goes for New Zealand, with its forty- to fifty-hour resident workweek. Total hours worked in every other

Western country remain below—sometimes far below—the United States, particularly in surgery.

Other countries have been able to reduce hours and improve working conditions more easily than in America for a variety of reasons. One is the nature of government-controlled health care, which can enact reforms more quickly and comprehensively than a fragmented private system if politicians sense an overwhelming public demand for change. Another possible explanation is the long-term emphasis beyond our borders on primary care. This has kept the number of specialists down to fifty percent in Britain, Canada, and other western nations; concurrently, the training tends to be less dominated by inpatient, specialized around-the-clock care.

Beyond this, physicians abroad lack the high degree of autonomy common to American physicians, medically and professionally but also culturally, a prediliction that in some cases has led U.S. doctors to arrogantly dismiss ideas and practices from other countries. For instance, some physicians in Britain argued as vociferously against reducing hours as opponents in the States, but now that Parliament has passed its decree, there is a powerful expectation among physicians that the rules will be obeyed. "The public has spoken," says Stern, sipping his tea in front of a large window in one of St. Thomas's meeting rooms. Behind him, out a large window, an early morning sun drenches the busy spires and ornaments of Parliament in golden light. "It is not our place to dig in and say we won't do it. I consider fifty-six hours a great challenge, to make it work. But it's got to be done."

■

In the United States, it is unlikely Congress will ever consider, much less pass, national rules of this sort for training physicians. States, too, have shelved plans to enact residency rules, in part because of the experience in New York state, where educators continue to chafe under the Bell Regulations, even as the program's success or failure remains unclear. Indeed, one suspects that short of assigning units of "reform police" in every ward, ICU, and O.R. in the Empire State, as long as educators fundamentally oppose reform, they will resist it unless it can be proven to be necessary.

Nor can we expect the ACGME's current approach to enforce change, though accreditors could strengthen their rules. They also need to enact effective enforcement mechanisms—including a system for legitimate individual grievances to be heard by impartial outside judges, and an authority to compel redress, if indicated. For their part, residents must continue to organize and call for change—with organized medicine protecting them from summary firings and abuse when they do.

Beyond this, the impetus for reform lingers where it has been since William Osler's day: with individual chiefs of service, program directors, and, to a lesser extent, hospitals. As Edmund Pellegrino suggested to me, the system rests on the idea of character—of individual chiefs, attendings, and residents knowing the difference between right and wrong. "The strongest way to teach virtue," he says, "is by example of someone they admire." This starts with the chairman of the department, he says, who must "focus responsibility" on doing the right thing. "Ethics also means being a big boy or girl," he adds. "I expect residents to be responsible, and to stay clear of what is right and wrong." This, he contends, is the best system of rules and enforcement.

Of course, Pellegrino is right. The problem is that this fervent hope of good triumphing in the end has not always worked.

■

This leaves us with what I consider two fundamental flaws in the reform process. First is the lack of data to prove (or disprove) the case for reform; which has led to the second—that educators without persuasive data are free to resist reform. And they will persist in doing so, even if every state in the United States passed Bell-style laws tomorrow, or a British-style fifty-six-hour week. As Timothy McCall wrote in 1989: "Residency reform will not be painless." In that spirit, I offer the following suggestions for reform—based on extensive conversations with educators, attendings, residents, health officials, ethicists, and patients.

To start with, physicians should confront the notion that they are *not* macho lawyers or Wall Street futures traders whose swagger, fatigue, and burnout hurts no one but themselves—and possibly their clients' wallets. It's time to change the mentality from one where being the ironman or ironwoman overrides all else, where instead a physician feels it his or her duty to say: "I will not operate for the fourth time today, because I am not at my best."

This reminds me of the senior resident who suggested that what doctors really need to do is all take a weekend off to sleep—if somehow the flow of patients could be stemmed for forty-eight hours. "What would happen if we all woke up rested and relaxed?" this resident asked. "Would we all realize what we are missing?"

A few specific suggestions:

1. Medicine should collect meaningful data on whether or not the current system is safe for patients and residents.

Americans spend billions of dollars ensuring that airplanes, roads, and automobiles are safe and that those who operate and maintain them are making as few errors as humanly possible. So it seems reasonable that medicine should embark on an immediate, serious effort to: (1) study the prevalence of residents' errors, how they happen, and how many are preventable—and how to amend the system to reduce errors; (2) settle once and for all the issue of fatigue—does it impair residents? How many hours can a resident work without becoming overly fatigued? Is fatigue dangerous? and (3) determine the optimal level of supervision, with experiments ranging from minimal to maximum vigilance by attendings, measuring the impact on education through proficiency tests, and on patient mortality and morbidity. These studies should be based on hard data and properly controlled experiments, not on surveys and other "soft" information.

I'm not exactly calling for the equivalent of the human genome project, though it's clear that reform will never happen until solid, indisputable information is gathered for those unwilling to accept common sense or the norm in other fields. Indeed, if proponents of the current system are so sure they are right, they could easily silence their critics by proving it with the same vigor they go after, say, a new drug to break up plaque in blood vessels, or teasing out which gene causes a rare blood disorder.

2. Abolish the traditional on-call system.

As Al Most noted, it makes little sense to jam a resident's schedule into one long, grueling day a week. From a human standpoint, it can be a bruising ordeal for the resident, and a disservice to patients whose doctors have too little time for them beyond their electrolyte counts and BUN. At worst, it's dangerous.

At the very least, programs should immediately institute a night-float system, with caps on the number of admissions—methods that have been used successfully for a half-century, and are a minimal first step toward implementing a Rhode Island–style no-call system. Another interim measure is protected sleep time for residents—a period of time when they are required to sleep (like airline pilots and naval officers), and will not be interrupted by beepers except in extreme emergencies.

Programs should develop their own version of a no-call system—wherein interns and residents admit one or two patients a day with a maximum of, say, seven a week, and go home each day when they have finished their work. Night and weekend floats would cover off hours. Safeguards must be built in to ensure they *do* go home—with the medical culture acknowledging the detriment to good care when doctors are overly fatigued, period.

For educators worried about continuity of care, and following the progression of diseases, treatments, and what happens post-op, this aspect of training should be consciously built into the system, with perhaps a "continuity block" where residents' only duty during that month is to track closely a few long-term patients. If a specific case requires them to stay up all night (it won't, in many instances), this should be a concentrated period when continuity is the object of the lesson, instead of the current arrangement, where residents sojourn in-house every second, third, or fourth night on the off chance a true continuity-of-care lesson *might* randomly occur.*

3. Teach residents how to hand off patients properly, and to work as teams.

After their training, physicians seldom stay at a single patient's bedside twenty-four hours a day—or for thirty-six hours every third or fourth day. According to a study authored by researchers at Harvard and The New York Hospital, a major complaint among attendings about New York's Bell laws is that residents must pass off patients more—and that the hands-offs are performed poorly. The study blamed this flaw on the rules, since fewer hours necessitates a higher turnover rate of residents vis-à-vis patients. But it's just as likely the residents in this study were not properly instructed in

---

*Surgeons more than nonsurgeons have a legitimate need to follow patients they have operated on, and should not be required to leave these patients by an arbitrary set of rules. However, most surgical interns and junior residents don't stay up all night sitting beside their post-op patients (neither do most attendings). Mostly, they are up doing scut work, and performing routine, patient-related tasks.

how to communicate vital information to other team members and night floats. I have observed dozens of "hand-offs." Typically, the information is imparted quickly, with no official form or procedures. At best, an intern heading home finds a quiet place to explain particulars about his or her patients to the person coming on duty. Sometimes, if it's busy, this meeting lasts only a few minutes and involves a quick, cursory exchange of key points and vitals.

Designing strong teams is essential to lessening hours—teams that resemble partnership systems among attendings and physicians out in the community, who spend their careers monitoring one another's patients, and jumping in if their colleague is unavailable. This means setting up systems to be sure residents share information about their patients, so that one team member can smoothly take over for another.

4. Attendings should be the primary teacher of residents and medical students.

There should be a corps of attending physicians assigned to teach and closely supervise residents in a hands-on, proactive manner, with an experienced senior physician awake and actively engaged on every service at all times. The goal would be to push trainees to excel, as Jennifer Jeremiah does, but in a more controlled, individual way than the current plunge-in method. This will cost money to train and hire more physician-teachers, but safety never comes cheaply, whether we are talking about air travel, highways, or patient care. Some of the costs will be mitigated by fewer costly errors. Likewise, residents should not be the primary teachers of residents one or two years below them, and interns should not be the primary teachers of medical students rotating through the wards. It is time to stop defending a system designed as much for convenience and economic reasons as for education, where researcher-clinician-administrators too often marginalize the process of true teaching and mentoring the residency was founded on—and fail to reward those who try to put teaching first.

5. Every major procedure and diagnosis should be formally taught and credentialed before a resident is allowed to perform it alone on a patient.

Most of the nondrug errors I witnessed involved mechanical procedures that can and should be taught, such as inserting arterial lines, intubating, and basic surgical procedures. The see one, do one, teach one model will not suffice in a high-tech era of medicine, even for low-tech operations. Already, some programs require residents to carry cards keeping track of how many procedures they have done; some further require a certain number before being certified. In the O.R., attending surgeons routinely evaluate residents, and require a certain mastery before allowing them to make the next cut. Even this system, however, depends on the individual attending, and almost never extends to procedures such as intubation that a resident is expected to perform on the surgical wards, often without supervision.

6. Improve working conditions and reform resident financing.

It's one thing to argue that residents must work ninety or a hundred hours to be properly educated. It's quite another if they are becoming dangerously exhausted because they are staying up to do scut, merely to save the hospital a few dollars, and to cover for attendings busy elsewhere. This is the 20 percent solution—to abolish the one-in-five hours residents spend performing scut, and prune back hours appropriately.

Also, resident pay should be linked (1) to what the market will bear in a competitive environment, which is what happens when residents moonlight; and (2) closer to the income residents bring in performing billable services, less what it costs to educate them. This means PGY5s would make considerably more than PGY1s—which is similar to what happens in every other profession, where junior associates and executives begin at a relatively low salary. Though most people already believe doctors are paid too much, residents are actually making less in real terms than the barely minimum wage salaries they earned in 1970—adding significantly to stress and to the sense that they deserve a big salary when they finish.

As salaries drop for physicians in general, and many more residents train for comparatively low wage positions in primary care, the issue of medical school costs and debt must also be seriously reconsidered. Indeed, more than ever, young physicians fresh out of residency are going to be finding themselves owing $100,000 and earning $80,000. Linking the pay of senior residents more closely to their service and skill levels will alleviate the stress of making ends meet in the face of hefty loan payments.

Of course, there is a palpable danger as managed care restructures residency financing, and teaching hospitals struggle to survive, that residency pay will decline, or that a "downsizing" of the number of residents will occur without adding ancillary backup, forcing trainees to take on even more scut than today. To avoid both hazards, hospitals and the health care community should once and for all determine how much is spent on educating physicians, how much of this is needed, and what society wants to spend. Once this is known, policymakers will be able to determine a stable method for financing medical education—whether it is a tax charged to all health care payers, further government subsidies, or something else.

7. Give residents responsibility more gradually.

Rather than plunge into a ward full of patients on day one, residents should ease into taking care of patients, working their way up to handling an entire ward. In fact, the original concept of the medical school clerkship in William Osler's day was to start trainees off with one patient at a time—still the norm today, though as suggested earlier, the teacher is usually an intern. Bertrand Bell's proposal to delay the awarding of the M.D. until during or after the residency might reinforce the reality that young physicians are not truly doctors when they graduate from medical school.

8. Teach and practice compassion—and much more.

It is not enough to teach a few hours of ethics, and the doctor-patient relationship, in the first year or two of medical school. Residents must see attendings and role models practicing empathy. Those teaching ethics should also emphasize that the practicality of kindness in many cases helps patients recover more quickly. Medical schools and residency programs would also be foolish to continue to ignore teaching finance, management, and health care policy, particularly in a managed-care era where physicians are required to be businesspeople as well as healers.

9. Get residents out of the wards.

One of the few truly revolutionary reforms of the past few years is the movement to pluck residents from the cloister of the hospital, where they treat only the most seriously ill patients, and out into "real life" situations: clinics, private doctors' offices, and

HMO offices. This should be greatly expanded, from the current 20 percent out-of-ward experience to 50 percent.

■

Even as I write these recommendations, the maelstrom of managed care is upon us—and with it potentially profound changes in graduate medical education.

Last year, the *New York Times* ran a leading editorial headlined "The Assault on Teaching Hospitals." It lambasted a new sort of triple threat to academic centers: the sizable cuts then being proposed by Congress in Medicare's funding of teaching programs; equally hefty cuts in medical research; and what the *Times* writers call the "dagger aimed at teaching hospitals" coming from private insurers and businesses that provide health coverage for their workers.

The *Times* goes on to say that teaching hospitals are "riddled with waste and turn out the wrong kind of doctors," and need to be downsized and the training made more relevant. "But these truths do not justify a mindless assault that threatens to bury the programs that turn out the best-trained physicians in the world." Much of the reform I've talked about in this chapter is threatened by the radical, wholesale change in the medical marketplace, which has abruptly relegated teaching hospitals from the crown jewels of America's health care system to what one managed care expert on Wall Street told me were "overpriced dinosaurs about to become extinct."

Already, there are warning signs of what may be coming ahead:

- The for-profit Timberlawn Psychiatric Hospital in Dallas canceled its residency program in 1993 and dismissed its trainees when managed care payers stopped paying for services rendered by junior physicians, reportedly because major employers in the area did not want their employers treated by trainees. Because Timberlawn's training program was funded almost entirely by patient revenues, they were forced to close it down—and according to a spokesman, regretted having to do so.
- Trying to save money as managed care contracts increase and revenues drop, Long Island Jewish Medical Center in Queens, New York, replaced a mostly private anesthesi-

ology service with a staff of younger, less costly—and less experienced—doctors. The state is now investigating several deaths on routine, usually nonfatal cases, one involving a resident who rapidly infused too much potassium into a fifty-year-old woman while she was undergoing intestinal surgery. (Potassium is usually infused slowly and in small doses, because too much can cause irregular heartbeats and cardiac arrest. The woman coded and died.) A hospital spokesperson told the *New York Times* that these were isolated cases, and that there are "no apparent quality of care issues" in the state's preliminary report on two of the episodes. Yet the ACGME specialty board for anesthesiology has put Long Island's program on probation, and the state continues to investigate.

Across the country, academic hospitals are struggling as managed care bypasses them for less expensive nonteaching hospitals, leaving many downtown facilities with a patient base that's increasingly composed of the indigent, the uninsured, and the elderly on Medicare, which pays just slightly more than managed care on average. In New York City, for instance, Columbia Presbyterian Hospital, long considered one of the best facilities in the Northeast, has amassed huge deficits as HMOs send patients elsewhere. Residents there complain that scut work is increasing, and that patient volume is down in some programs to the point that there are too few to go around for a proper education.

In Boston, Brigham and Women's and Massachusetts General last year announced plans to cut their number of residents by as much as 15 percent over the next few years. In 1995, they cut 5 percent, eliminating 20 slots out of 360; in 1996 they plan to cut another 30 to 50 slots. This was in anticipation of Congress's slicing Medicare payments, and steep reductions in payments by managed care companies to teaching hospitals in the Boston area. In California, Los Angeles County Hospital, which is currently training hundreds of residents, was in danger last year of being closed down as the county's health care department faces a $650 million deficit in a $2.5 billion health care budget—a shortfall caused because of dramatic increases in numbers of uninsured patients, and steep reductions in revenues as managed care dominates the southern California health care market.

Some teaching hospitals are fighting back to counter what many consider a medical market that seems less than sympathetic to teaching. For instance, in Boston, Harvard Medical School and Beth Israel Hospital recently formed a new joint venture to shift attention back to teaching—and to study ways to restructure the financing and curriculum of education given the new realities of medicine. In a statement announcing the new program, physician-educators at Beth Israel warned that "the bottom line" was imperiling medical education, and that they hoped to "counteract this trend, balancing the intensifying business pressures with a renewed emphasis on the academic mission . . ."

Yet it follows that if teaching hospitals are closing and under siege, residency reform may become a casualty—particularly if the studies I'm calling for do show patients are more at risk in teaching hospitals than nonteaching facilities.

Still, I believe that Congress and the public will intervene long before teaching hospitals are driven out of business. The simple logic of needing to train a reasonable number of future physicians—and of keeping valuable and popular research on line—is overwhelming. It's even conceivable that when it comes time to reorganize funding for teaching centers in a comprehensive way, the system will be shaken up to the point that more reform will be possible. It's also conceivable that managed care will *force* significant reform when—and if—a true consumer-oriented quality of care dynamic takes hold in medicine, as it has for automobiles, dishwashers, and tennis racquets. Indeed, there is a nascent movement afoot to acquire and to organize sophisticated outcomes data, which may make it possible in the near future to truly compare quality of care in hospitals.

But what if fair, balanced outcomes indicate that teaching hospitals *are* more dangerous than they should be? And what if even further refinements in outcomes data suggest that the residency *system* is to blame and needs to be overhauled? Of course, it's possible that real outcomes data will prove teaching hospitals are, in fact, safe. If this fails to happen, however, a poor report card may force programs to change how they teach physicians—but not in the gradual, more thoughtful way that is still feasible now. In fact, it might serve academic hospitals well to counter the antiresident attitude that closed Timberlawn's program by quickly instituting residency reforms in the name of improving quality of care.

Whatever the outcome of the current flux, this is certainly no time to ignore reforms—or what the public wants, and managed care providers may demand. Nor is it the time to be trying to maintain a status quo and tradition that is increasingly indefensible—and continues to belie common sense.

A Photograph of Michael

at the Ending of this road,
a candle in a shrine:

e. e. cummings

Not long ago, a small photograph appeared on my kitchen table. Only an inch square, it showed a baby a few months old. He was smiling, and wearing what looked like a little infant sailor suit. I asked my physician-wife where it came from, and she grew quiet. "That's Michael," she said, a baby she had struggled to save when he was born with a congenital heart defect. "They gave out this little picture at the funeral," which she had attended that day.

She studied the tiny picture, and said nothing—which is her way. But I knew what she was thinking; that this was a little boy like our own children, one she had tried hard to keep alive, but couldn't. She had also greatly admired Michael's parents, who tried everything, but in the end let go of their little baby when they knew all hope was lost.

As I watched her gazing at the smiling baby, I understood all over again why my wife went into medicine—and why she was willing to suffer through her training.

It was because of this little boy.

This was also why Jim Stern probably cried that night during Mary Allen's ordeal, and why Rich Ferrara was infuriated by what happened in the O.R. to the woman with the back injury. It was also why Carol Tisch was so upset at having to make a choice, as she saw it, between her values and being a surgeon.

This is the reason medicine is not like making automobiles, or flying an airplane, or being in the Marines, and should never be subsumed by function at the expense of form.

■

At the moment, it's popular to complain about escalating crime, declining family values, and so forth, but all this really means is that we as a society, including physicians, are desperately searching for anchors; for something to help us make sense of things. This is why it's so critical to understand that people need healers, and that healers need people. As Tom Delbanco might say, there is a scientific side to medicine, and a spiritual side—a time for cutting and diagnosis, and a time for magic.

We need more magic, I think, on the wards and in the O.R.'s. For Michael's sake. And Mary Allen's, and for all the rest of us.

Unless otherwise indicated, all quotes in the text were acquired during interviews or in the field by the author. Most interviews were either tape-recorded or transcribed in a notebook. In most cases, the dialogue, action, and facts were checked by phone or in person with major subjects. The author allowed subjects to propose minor alterations to conversations to clarify points or to protect sources, though nothing originally spoken was changed substantially. A few subjects did not respond when called to verify quotes, despite repeated attempts. In a very few instances, the author was forced to depend on his memory to recall conversations and events. These were verified later with the subject, when possible.

7 Opening Epigram. *we teach Physicians:* John Stobo spoke these words during an interview in 1991. When they were read back to him in 1995, he said he still agreed with the statement.

FOREWORD: A LONG, COLD WINTER

15 Epigram. *in all things:* William Shakespeare, *King Henry V, The Complete Works* (Secaucus, NJ: Wellfleet Press, 1987), Act V, scene 1, p. 851.

18 *burn [with passion]:* E. Frank, "On Burning," letter, *The Journal of the American Medical Society (JAMA),* Vol. 261 (1989), p. 1980.

18 *and garage mechanics:* From a poll taken on April 18, 1995. Source: the Roper Center at the University of Connecticut, Public Opinion Online.

21 *almost 100,000 residents:* See *Annual Report,* Accreditation Council for Graduate Medical Education (1994), p. 3.

21 *7200 residency programs:* Ibid.

21 *1200 teaching hospitals:* See *Hospital Statistics,* American Hospital Association (1993–1994), p. 200.

PROLOGUE: 3 I HOURS

22 *Stern is furious:* All names in the prologue are pseudonyms, at the subjects' request. The use of pseudonyms in this book is regrettable, though it does help to reinforce the author's intention to focus on the issues, not on persons or specific institutions.

27 *a single night:* N. Lurie, et al., "How Do House Officers Spend Their Nights? A Time Study of Internal Medicine House Staff on Call," *The New England Journal of Medicine (NEJM)* (1989), pp. 1673–1677. Also see Connie Parenti, et. al., "Are Things Different in the Light of Day? A Time Study of Internal Medicine House Staff Days," *The American Journal of Medicine,* Volume 94 (June, 1993), pp. 654–658.

32 *included Mary Allen:* Jim Stern did not agree with using the term "error" to describe the Mary Allen episode, preferring to call it an "unfortunate incident."

CHAPTER I: MEANS TO AN END

35 Epigram. *as means only:* Immanuel Kant, "Good Will, Duty and the Categorical Imperative," *Fundamental Principles of Metaphysics of Morals.,* Sec. 1 and 2 (New York: Abbott, 1898), p. 17.

37 *do not lie!:* Fyodor Mikhailovich Dostoyevsky, *The Brothers Karamazov,* trans. David Magarshack (New York: Penguin Books, 1987), p. 287. This question was posed by Ivan Karamazov to his brother, Alyosha, who answered: "No, I wouldn't."

37 *(or resident) error:* More and more, data on quality and outcomes is being collected by insurance and government agencies, though this information has yet to be analyzed in a meaningful, easily understood format, or to be integrated into widespread daily medical practice. See Lawrence K. Altman, "Medical Errors Bring Calls for Change," *New York Times,* July 18, 1995, p. C1.

39 *mistakes are inevitable:* Lucian Leape, "Error in Medicine," *JAMA,* 272:23 (December 21, 1994), p. 1852.

39 *(in a hospital):* Ibid., p. 1851. The figure of 180,000 deaths is extrapolated from a 1991 study authored by Leape and several colleagues, who took data on adverse medical events in New

York State and analyzed it to determine how many of the cases involved error. According to that study, nearly 4% of all New York patients received an injury that either prolonged their hospital stay, or resulted in a "measurable disability." Nearly 14% of these injuries were fatal, according to the study. See T.A. Brennan et. al., "Incidence of Adverse Events and Negligence in Hospitalized Patients: Results of the Harvard Medical Practice Study I," *NEJM*, Vol. 324 (1991), pp. 370–376; and Leape et. al., "Incidence of Adverse Events and Negligence in Hospitalized Patients: Results of the Harvard Medical Practice Study II," *NEJM*, Volume 324 (1991), pp. 377–384.

39 *therefore, potentially preventable:* Lucian Leape, "Error in Medicine," p. 1851.

39 *studied in 1991:* See T.A. Brennan et. al., "Incidence of Adverse Events . . . the Harvard Medical Practice Study I," pp. 370–376; and Leape et al., "Incidence of Adverse Events . . . the Harvard Medical Practice Study II," pp. 377–384.

39 *every two days:* Lucian Leape, "Error in Medicine," p. 1851.

39 *substandard medical care:* Michelle White, "The Value of Liability in Medical Malpractice," *Health Affairs*, 13:4 (Fall, 1994). Also see P. Danzon, *Medical Malpractice: Theory, Evidence, and Public Policy* (Cambridge, MA: Harvard University Press, 1985); M.I. Taragin et. al., "The Influence of Standard of Care and Severity of Injury on the Resolution of Medical Malpractice Claims," *Annals of Internal Medicine*, Volume 117 (1992), pp. 780–784.

39 *resulting in death:* See *Annual Report*, Hospital Incident Reporting Program, New York Department Of Health (1989), p. 7.

39 *of medical errors:* The figure of 45,000 deaths was determined by taking total hospital admissions in the U.S. for 1989, i.e., 25 million (source: AHA statistics, 1993–94, p. XI), and calculating it against the deaths due to hospital-caused adverse events per thousand patients discharged from New York state hospitals, as reported in New York State's Incident Report for 1989. The rate as reported was .18 per 1000 discharges. See *Annual Report*, Hospital Incident Reporting Program, New York Department Of Health (1989), p. 7.

39 *motor vehicle accidents:* Source for airline fatalities: National Transportation Safety Board; source for motor vehicle accidents: National Safety Council. See *The World Almanac*, ed. Robert Famighetti (Mahwah, NJ: World Almanac, 1995), pp. 296, 964.

40 *teaching programs (3.4%):* Troyen A. Brennan et. al., "Hospital Characteristics Associated With Adverse Events and Substandard Care," *JAMA,* 265:24 (June 26, 1991), pp. 3265–3269.

41 *percent who died:* Albert W. Wu, et.al., "Do House Officers Learn from Their Mistakes?" *JAMA,* 265:16 (April 24, 1991), pp. 2089–94.

41 *1,000 for attendings:* Timothy S. Lesar et. al., "Medication Prescribing Errors in a Teaching Hospital," *JAMA,* 263:17 (May 2, 1990), pp. 2329–2334.

41 *a single month:* This study was given to me by a resident in the hospital where the survey of house staff errors was conducted. He asked that his identity and that of the hospital be kept confidential.

41 *by the state:* Lisa Belkin, "Tracking Medical Errors, From Humans to Machines," *New York Times,* March 31, 1992.

41 *to the brain:* Ibid. State investigators verified the essential facts in Belkin's article. They also directed me to a passage in their department's 1989 Incidents Report, which reads: "The substantial number and percentage of deaths and other serious incidents in which house staff and postgraduate trainees are involved are of particular concern." According to the report, residents contributed to 60 verified deaths in New York in 1989—and to hundreds of injuries. See *Annual Report,* Hospital Incident Reporting Program, New York Department Of Health, 1989.

41 *a hernia operation:* Ibid.

41 *attendings and nurses:* Ibid.

43 *almost free care:* For a good overview of the recent history of medical education, the residency, and medicine in general in America and Europe, start with the following: Charles E. Rosenberg, *The Care of Strangers: The Rise of America's Hospital System* (New York: Basic Books, 1987); Kenneth M. Ludmerer, *Learning to Heal: The Development of American Medical Education* (New York: Basic Books, 1985); Paul Starr, *The Social Transformation of American Medicine* (New York: Basic Books, 1982); William G. Rothstein, *American Physicians in the Nineteenth Century: From Sects to Science* (Baltimore: The Johns Hopkins University Press, 1985) and *American Medical School and the Practice of Medicine* (Oxford: Oxford University Press); ed. Judith Leavitt and Ronald L. Numbers, *Sickness and Health*

in America: Readings in the History of Medicine and Public Health (Madison, WI: The University of Wisconsin Press 1985); and John Duffy, *From Humors to Medical Science: A History of American Medicine* (Urbana, IL: University of Illinois Press, 1993). Parts of the historic sections of this book are also based on two phone conversations with medical historian and sociologist William Rothstein of the University of Maryland at Baltimore.

46 *seems to deserve:* John F. Christensen, et. al., "The Heart of Darkness: The Impact of Perceived Mistakes on Physicians," *Journal of General Internal Medicine,* Volume 7 (July/August, 1992), p. 424.

47 *of an M&M:* Leape insists that all obvious errors at the hospitals and departments in which he has worked have always been discussed at M&M's. Given the sheer numbers cited in his and other studies, time constraints suggest that this would be difficult, though perhaps not impossible.

47 *Charles L. Bosk:* Charles L. Bosk, *Forgive and Remember: Managing Medical Failure* (Chicago: The University of Chicago Press, 1979), p. 3–4.

47 *and not repeated:* Ibid.

47 *for a patient:* Ibid, p. 40.

48 *mistakes are inevitable:* Leape, "Errors in Medicine," p. 1852.

CHAPTER 2: THE PLUNGE-IN METHOD

51 Epigram. *mastery and growth:* Abraham Flexner, quoted by Edmund Pellegrino in his essay, "The Reconciliation of Technology and Humanism," *Flexner: Seventy-five Years Later,* ed. Charles Vevier (Lanham, MD: University Press of America, 1987), p. 105.

51 *as an intern:* All names in the surgical trauma sequence are pseudonyms, with the exception of Tom Kirsch.

58 *"hard to know."* Kidd didn't explain, however, how running a tube into the stomach would have told them anything about the spleen. "They aren't connected," said Hopkins' Tom Kirsch. "You don't want an NG tube for that, anyway. You want a CT or a DPL." A DPL is a Diagnostic Peritoneal Lavage. In this procedure, one injects saline into the abdominal cavity and then withdraws it to check for internal bleeding.

59 *and of rashness:* From the "Law" section of the *Hippocratic Corpus,* c. fourth and fifth centuries, B.C.; quoted from *Ethics in Medicine: Historic Perspectives and Contemporary Concerns,* ed. Stanley Joel Riser, et. al. (Cambridge, MA: MIT Press, 1977), p. 8. The *Hippocratic Corpus* is a collection of documents that have survived from what scholars call the Hippocratic school of medicine, in existence during the fifth to fourth centuries, B.C., in ancient Greece. Hippocrates himself was born in 460 B.C., on the island of Cos, and traveled and taught throughout the Greek world during a long life. Some of the *Corpus* may have been written by Hippocrates himself, though authorship of the documents remains unclear.

59 *treatment with safety:* Ibid.

59 *inexperience of physicians:* Frederick II, law for the regulation of medicine in the two Sicilies, 1240 or 1241; from James J. Walsh, *The Popes and Science: The History of the Papal Relations to Science During the Middle Ages and Down to Our Own Time* (New York: Fordham University Press, 1911), pp. 419–423.

59 *the poor patients:* Quoted from Edward Atwater, "Touching the Patient: The Teaching of Internal Medicine in America," in *Sickness and Health in America: Readings in the History of Medicine and Public Health,* Second Edition, ed. Judith Walzer Leavitt and Ronald L. Numbers (Madison, WI: The University of Wisconsin Press 1985), p. 133. This occurred in 1819, though as Atwater writes, "This feeling apparently still existed in 1846 when the managers [at Massachusetts General Hospital], responding to a proposal to move the medical school adjacent to the hospital, stated 'that they cannot perceive any advantage to this institution to arise therefrom.' "

60 *room and board:* See Paul Starr, *The Social Transformation of American Medicine* (New York: Basic Books, 1982), pp. 220–221, 358.

61 *farmers, and servants:* Plato, *The Republic;* from *Great Dialogues of Plato,* Book III, tr. W.H.D. Rouse (New York: New American Library, 1956), p. 215.

CHAPTER 3: A WORKING KNOWLEDGE

64 Epigram. *of the whole:* William Mayo, quoted in Helen Clapesattle, *The Doctors Mayo* (Minneapolis, MN: University of Minnesota Press, 1941), p. 530.

68 *drugs a year* (footnote): See Herrman Blumgardt, "Medicine: The Art and the Science," *On Doctoring*, ed. Richard Reynolds and John Stone (New York: Simon & Schuster, 1991), p. 108.

69 *the United States:* For information on numbers of residents and teaching hospitals in the U.S. in 1940 see Jonathon Klein, "Resident Education, Work Hours, and Supervision: Time for Change," *Journal of Pediatrics*, 116:3 (March, 1990), p. 484.

69 *almost 100,000 residents:* See *Annual Report*, Accreditation Council for Graduate Medical Education, 1994, p. 3.

69 *at 1,223 teaching hospitals:* See *Hospital Statistics*, American Hospital Association, 1993–4, p. 200.

69 *percent minorities today:* David Ewing Duncan, "Is This Any Way to Train a Doctor: Medical Residencies: The Next Health Care Crisis," *Harper's*, April 1993, 61–66.

69 *officers are married:* See Abraham Bergman, et. al., "Pediatric Resident's Working Hours," *Journal of Pediatrics*, 116:3 (March 1990), p. 479.

71 *at present levels:* Timothy McCall, "The Impact of Long Working Hours on Resident Physicians," *NEJM*, 318:12 (March 24, 1988), p. 777.

72 *careful clinical reasoning:* Jerome P. Kassirer, "Teaching Problem Solving—How Are We Doing?" *NEJM*, 332:22 (June 1, 1995), pp. 1507–1508.

CHAPTER 4: SIGNING OFF

74 *in the OR:* Rich Ferrera is a pseudonym.

78 *notes Geena Carlson:* Geena Carlson is a pseudonym.

80 *a single month:* At the request of the resident who provided this confidential study, the author is keeping the name of the hospital anonymous.

80 *and complication rates:* See William F. Fallon Jr., et al., "Resident Supervision in the Operating Room: Does This Impact on Outcome?" *The Journal of Trauma*, 35:4 (October, 1993), pp. 556–561.

81 *under strict supervision: Report of the Fourth Grand Jury for the April/May Term of 1986 Concerning the Care and Treatment of a Patient and the Supervision of Interns and Junior Residents at*

a Hospital in New York County, The New York Supreme Court, December 31, 1986, Preface, p. 4.

81 *postgraduate residency program:* Ibid.

82 *and expected demand:* The Final Report of the Ad Hoc Advisory Committee on Emergency Services (The Bell Commission), New York Department of Health, October, 1987, p. 3.

82 *in the OR:* See Testimony of Paul Ebert, *The Final Report of the Ad Hoc Advisory Committee on Emergency Services* (The Bell Commission).

82 *of mandatory rule:* See the various testimonies of physicians and medical groups transcribed in *The Final Report of the Ad Hoc Advisory Committee on Emergency Services* (The Bell Commission).

82 *to increase supervision:* John E. Albers, speaking for the American Medical Association, told the Bell Commission: "The AMA supports the goal of the Committee's recommendation that residents should receive adequate supervision. . . . However, implementation of the Committee's proposal would undoubtedly result in increased costs to teaching hospitals and greater time demands on supervising physicians." Testimony of John E. Albers, M.D., "Statement of the American Medical Association," August 17, 1987, *The Final Report of the Ad Hoc Advisory Committee on Emergency Services* (The Bell Commission).

82 *control, minimum interference:* Testimony of the American College of Physicians, August 17, 1987, *The Final Report of the Ad Hoc Advisory Committee on Emergency Services* (The Bell Commission).

83 *of their competence:* Ibid.

83 *some improper judgments:* Ibid.

83 *of the art:* From the "Decorum" section of the *Hippocratic Corpus,* c. fourth and fifth centuries, B.C.; quoted from Riser, *Ethics in Medicine,* p. 8.

84 *of the wards:* Ludmerer, *Learning to Heal,* pp. 68–69.

84 *principles of practice:* William Osler, "Farewell Address to the Johns Hopkins University," 1905, quoted in *Counsels and Ideals from the Writings of William Osler* (New York: Houghton, Mifflin & Company, 1905), p. 150.

84 *Mrs. Jones's ventilator:* For information about the increase in use of residents and the decline of attendings on the wards, see Starr, *The Social Transformation of American Medicine,* pp. 358, 360.

85 *visit Steve Jones:* Steve Jones is a pseudonym.

86 *(one to two):* See Paul Jolly, "Medical Education in the United States, 1960–1987," *Health Affairs,* 7:2 (Supplement, 1988), pp. 146, 149.

86 *with direct education:* The amount of time faculty spends with residents varies a great deal according to specialties, programs, hospitals, and individual attendings.

86 *percent with patients:* Steven Guarisco et. al., "Time Analysis of a General Medicine Service," *Journal of General Internal Medicine,* vol. 9 (May 1994), p. 275.

87 *extra per year:* Testimony of Jo Ivey Boufford, President, New York City Health and Hospitals Corporation, August 20, 1987. *The Final Report of the Ad Hoc Advisory Committee on Emergency Services* (The Bell Commission).

88 *meaningful mentoring experience:* For information on the crisis in mentoring, see Marilyn M. Schapira et. al., "Mentorship in General Internal Medicine," *Journal of Internal Medicine,* Volume 7 (March/April, 1992); for general information on mentoring, see D.J. Levinson, *The Seasons of a Man's Life,* (New York: Ballantine Books, 1978). Also see David Ewing Duncan, "The Gift of Wisdom," *Hippocrates,* Vol. 9, No. 1 (January, 1995), PP. 36–7. In recent years, some educators have sounded the alarm about the decline in mentoring, and have tried to counter the trend by encouraging close relationships between senior and junior physicians. One example is the Generalist Physician Faculty Scholar's Program, put in place by Steve Schroeder, President of the Robert Wood Johnson Foundation. This program offers substantial funding—up to $240,000 for a four-year grant—to young physicians to enable them to work closely with a mentor of their choice as they pursue a research topic.

89 *known as rigors:* See Testimony of Gregory Stone, *Zion vs. New York Hospital, Raymond Sherman, Luise Weinstein, Gregory Stone, and Maurice Leonard,* New York Supreme Court, November 10, 1994 to February 6, 1995.

89 *one been present:* Raymond Sherman, the attending in charge of the residents tending to Libby Zion the morning she died, testified that he was not told about the Demoral being administered. Had he been informed, he further testified, he would have told the residents not to use Demoral. See Testimony of Raymond Sherman,

Zion v. New York Hospital, New York Supreme Court, 1994–95.

89 *and killed her:* Libby Zion's father, Sidney Zion, his lawyers, and some medical experts theorized that the mix of Demoral and Nardil may have contributed to her illness and possibly to her death. The jury in *Zion v. New York Hospital* agreed, declaring the doctors negligent for administering Demoral, and finding that this contributed to Libby's "pain and suffering or death." See Verdict Sheet, *Zion v. New York Hospital,* dated February 6, 1995.

89 *year-old patient:* For the official record of this case, see "Statement of Deficiency and Plan of Correction," *Report by Albany Medical Center Hospital,* November 15, 1994, New York Department of Health, pp. 6–8.

90 *or attending physician:* Ibid., p. 8.

98 *Jim Stern's team:* Benjamin Frain is a pseudonym.

98 *Do it again:* The author thanks Dr. Robert Nye for sharing this story.

CHAPTER 5: BALM OF HURT MINDS

102 *frustrated Ben Rollins:* Ben Rollins is a pseudonym.

103 *five-day period:* Truly excessive on-call shifts are rarer today than they used to be, though they still occur in some programs. For instance, see Jonathon Klein, "Resident Education, Work Hours, and Supervision: Time for Change," *Journal of Pediatrics,* 116:3 (March, 1990), pp. 484–486. Klein cites studies documenting the fact that forty-eight to seventy-two-hour weekend calls are still the norm in some surgical programs. (Residents frequently get some sleep during these long in-house coverage shifts). Klein also mentions a surgical intensive care unit in Texas that assigns its residents to a rotation that is forty-five days straight, without a day off.

104 *patient care performance:* This study was provided to me with the understanding that the name of the institution would remain anonymous.

104 *of sleep deprivation:* For a brief history of sleep research in the 1890s see Heinz Schmidtke, "Disturbance of Processing of Information," Chapter 10 of *Psychological Aspects and Physiological*

Correlates of Work and Fatigue, ed. E. Jimonsoa and P. Neiser (Charles C. Thomas, 1976), p. 238. Merrill Mitler, director of sleep research at the Scripps Institute in La Jolla, California, also provided some historic information on fatigue during two phone interviews in the summer of 1995. Some of the first studies in sleep deprivation research were conducted in Germany. They include E. Amberg, "Über den Einfluß von Arbeitspausen auf die geistige Leistungsfähigkeit," *Psychol Arbeiten,* 1:300 (1896) and W.H.R. Rivers and E. Kraepelin, "Über Ermüdung und Erholung," *Psychol Arbeiten,* 1:627 (1896). It was German researcher G. Aschaffenburg who early on studied disturbances of thinking caused by fatigue, and associated it in 1899 with the pathology of "Ideenflucht," the "flight of ideas." See G. Aschaffenburg, "Experimentelle Studien über Assoziation II," *Psychol Arbeiten,* 2:1 (1899).

105 *and factory laborers:* This information comes from telephone interviews with Merrill Mitler, summer, 1995. Also see Mathew Wald, "FAA Wants to Cut Jetliner Pilots' Hours," *New York Times,* December 15, 1995, p. A35; Anastasia Toufexis, "Drowsy America," *Time,* December 17, 1990, pp. 85. For a sampling of the very extensive body of research on the detrimental effects of sleep deprivation in general, and specifically as it relates to different industries, see M. Anch, et. al., *Sleep: A Scientific Perspective,* (Englewood Cliffs, New Jersey: Prentice-Hall 1988); *Principals of Sleep Medicine,* ed. M.H. Kryger, et. al. (Philadelphia: W. B. Saunders, 1993); National Commission of Sleep Disorders Research, *Wake Up America: A National Sleep Alert,* Volume 1 (Bethesda, MD: National Institutes of Health January, 1993); studies include W.P. Colquhoun, et. al., "Work at Sea: A Study of Sleep, and of Circadian Rhythms in Physiological and Psychological Functions," *International Archives of Occupational and Environ Health,* Vol. 60, No. 5 (1988), pp. 321–329; Merrill Mitler, et. al., "When People Die: Cause of Death versus Time of Death," *The American Journal of Medicine,* Volume 82 (February, 1987); John K. Lauber and Phyllis J. Kayten, "Sleepiness, Circadian Dysrhythmia, and Fatigue in Transportation System Accidents," *Sleep,* 11 (6) (1988), pp. 503–512; John M. Taub, "Disturbances in Diurnal Rhythms Following a Night of Reduced Sleep," *International Journal of Neuroscience,* Volume

14 (1981), pp. 239–245; and D.R. Haslam, "Sleep loss, recovery sleep, and military performance," *Ergonomics*, Vol. 25, No. 2 (1982), pp. 163–178. There are hundreds more studies on virtually all aspects of this subject.

105 *to ten hours:* See Mathew Wald, "FAA Wants to Cut Jetliner Pilots' Hours," *New York Times*, December 15, 1995, p. A35.

105 *at the controls:* Anastasia Toufexis, "Drowsy America," *Time*, December 17, 1990, pp. 85. Merrill Mitler confirmed that the rules for pilots napping have been enacted by the FAA.

105 *every twenty-four:* Merrill Mitler, telephone interview.

105 *of . . . their units:* Quoted in "Report on the Center for Army Lessons Learned," *New York Times*, May 31, 1988, p. A17.

105 *accidents a year:* The U.S. Department of Transportation, as reported by Deborah L. Shelton, "Sleep-deprived Drivers Linked to Highway 'Carnage,' " *American Medical News*, July 17, 1995, p. 6.

105 *at its greatest:* Studies on circadian rhythms are extensive. For a popularly written appraisal, see Anastasia Toufexis, "Drowsy America," *Time*, December 17, 1990, p. 80; for a sampling of the research see *Biological Rhythms: Implications for the Worker*, U.S. Congress, Office of Technology Assessment, OTA-BA-463 (Washington, D.C.: U.S. Government Printing Office, September, 1991); Merrill Mitler et. al., "When People Die: Cause of Death versus Time of Death," *The American Journal of Medicine*, Volume 82 (February, 1987); John K. Lauber and Phyllis J. Kayten, "Sleepiness, Circadian Dysrhythmia, and Fatigue in Transportation System Accidents," *Sleep*, 11 (6) (1988), pp. 503–512; John M. Taub, "Disturbances in Diurnal Rhythms Following a Night of Reduced Sleep," *International Journal of Neuroscience*, Volume 14 (1981), pp. 239–245; W.P. Colquhoun et. al., "Work at Sea: Sleep and Circadian Rhythms in Watchkeepers," *International Archives of Occupational and Environmental Health*, 60 (1988), pp. 321–329. This is by no means an exhaustive list.

106 *movements at rest:* For examples, see John Robbins and Fred Gottlieb, "Sleep Deprivation and Cognitive Testing in Internal Medicine House Staff," *The Western Journal of Medicine*, 152:1 (January, 1990), pp. 82–8; C.H.M. Jacques et. al., "The Effects of Sleep Loss on Cognitive Performance of Resident Physicians,"

The Journal of Family Practice, Vol. 30, No. 2 (1990), pp. 223–229; Gary S. Richardson, "Objective Assessment of Sleep and Alertness in Medical House-Staff and the Impact of Protected Time for Sleep" (1992). Available from Dr. Richardson at Brigham and Women's Hospital, Boston; Rachel Rubin et. al., "Neurobehavioral Effects of the On-Call Experience in House-Staff Physicians," *Journal of Occupational Medicine,* Vol. 33, No. 1 (January, 1991); Richard Denisco, et. al., "The Effect of Fatigue on the Performance of a Simulated Anesthetic Monitoring Task," *Journal of Clinical Monitoring,* Vol. 3, No. 1 (January, 1987); D.I. Orton and J.H. Gruzelier, "Adverse Changes in Mood and Cognitive Performance of House Officers after Night Duty," *British Medical Journal,* 298 (1989), 23–26. This is by no means an exhaustive list.

106 *of hurt minds:* William Shakespeare, *Macbeth* (II, i, 62).

108 *room from exhaustion:* From *Bad Medicine?,* a documentary film produced and directed in 1994 by three students at the Columbia School of Journalism: Geralyn Lucas, Sloane Karron, and Diane Morril. Lucas is married to a surgical resident.

108 *one forty-five:* Joseph Berger, "The Long Days and Short Life of a Third-Year Medical Student," *The New York Times,* May 30, 1993.

109 *the general population:* The true suicide rate among physicians remains elusive, with surveys and extrapolations providing a range from 31 per 100,000 doctors to 88 per 100,000, though most experts tend to side with the lower number. This compares to about 12 per 100,000 for the general population. For white males over twenty-five, the rate is 31 out of 100,000. For information on suicide among physicians and the general public, see Council on Scientific Affairs, "Results and Implications of the AMA-APA Physician Mortality Project," *JAMA,* Vol. 257, No. 21 (June 5, 1987); Report by the U.S. Centers for Disease Control and Prevention, "Youth Suicide Rates, 1950–90," *Morbidity and Mortality Weekly Report* (April 22, 1994); Betty Hosmer Mawardi, "Satisfactions, Dissatisfactions, and Causes of Stress in Medical Practice," *JAMA,* Vol. 241, No. 14 (April 6, 1979); Jack D. McCue, "Effects of Stress on Physicians and Their Medical Practice," *NEJM,* (February 25, 1982); M. Olkinuora et. al., "Stress Symptoms, Burnout and Suicidal Thoughts in Finnish Physi-

cians," *Social Psychiatry and Psychiatric Epidemiology* (1990); Ralph Cranshaw et. al., "An Epidemic of Suicide Among Physicians on Probation," *JAMA*, Vol. 243, No. 119 (May 16, 1980).

109 *the general population:* Like suicide, data on the extent of substance abuse among physicians is sketchy at best. Estimates have ranged from a rate of abuse that is equal to or slightly above the general population to as much as thirty times the rate of the general population, a number that is almost certainly too high, according to some experts. For information on physician substance abuse, see David I. Canavan, "The Subject of Impairment," Journal of the Medical Society of New Jersey, Vol. 80, No. 1 (1983), pp. 47–48; W.A. Spickard, "Impaired Physician," Alcoholism: A Guide for the Primary Care, (Abstract), ed. M. Lipkin, et. al. (New York: Springer-Verlag, 1988), p. 5; Patrick H. Hughes et. al., "Prevalence of Substance Use Among U.S. Physicians," *JAMA*, Vol. 267, No. 17 (May 6, 1992); Richard D. Aach, et. al., "Alcohol and Other Substance Abuse and Impairment Among Physicians in Residency Training," *Annals of Internal Medicine*, Vol. 116 (1992), p. 245; David L. Schiedermayer and Bonnie J. Tesch, "Primary Care Physician Burnout: Definitions, Self-Assessment and Treatment," *Wisconsin Medical Journal* (April 1992), pp. 179–182; Stephen C. Mason, "How the MSMS Impaired Physician Program Works," *Michigan Medicine* (May 1982); Jack D. McCue, "Effects of Stress on Physicians and Their Medical Practice," *NEJM* (February 25, 1982); and Patrick H. Hughes "Resident Physician Substance Use in the United States," *JAMA*, Vol. 265, No. 16 (April 24, 1991).

109 *marriages and relationships:* Psychiatrists and marriage experts say that physicians are at high risk for divorce and marital problems. For example, see Jack D. McCue, "Effects of Stress on Physicians and Their Medical Practice," *NEJM* (February 25, 1982).

109 *while on duty:* Steven Daugherty, et. al., "Survey of Resident Educational and Working Conditions," *Report to the AMA-ERF* (Chicago: American Medical Association, April, 1991).

111 *cause of errors:* See Albert W. Wu, et. al., "Do House Officers Learn from Their Mistakes?" *JAMA*, 265:16 (April 24, 1991), pp. 2089–94. Residents in this survey in most cases attributed adverse outcomes to multiple causes. This is why the percentages don't equal 100 percent.

112 onto the patient: Anastasia Toufexis, "Drowsy America," p. 80.

112 prescribed another medication: Ibid.

113 while on call: Timothy McCall, "The Impact of Long Working Hours on Resident Physicians," *NEJM*, 318:12 (March 24, 1988), p. 776.

114 difficult to manage: Colford and McPhee identify a "House Officer Syndrome" brought on by stress, fatigue, and the sudden immersion into the responsibility of taking care of very sick patients; one of the outgrowths of the syndrome is residents' cynicism and even an active dislike of some of their patients. See J.M. Colford and S.J. McPhee, "The Ravelled Sleeve of Care—Managing the Stress of Residency Training," *JAMA*, 261 (1989), pp. 889–893. Also see Catherine A. Martin and Rachel A. Julian, "Causes of Stress and Burnout in Physicians Caring for the Chronically and Terminally Ill," ed. Lenora Finn, *Stress and Burnout Among Providers Caring for the Terminally Ill and Their Families* (Paradis, N.Y.: Haworth Press, 1987), pp. 121–146. Dr. Nassir Ghaemi, a psychiatrist at the Medical College of Virginia, provided personal observations and perspectives as someone who has treated residents for depression and other psychological maladies.

114 lizard, and reeker: Victoria George and Alan Dundes, "The Gomer: A Figure of American Folk Speech." I have been unable to pinpoint the source of this excellent chapter from a book, which was given to me without citation. Apparently, George and Dundes hail from the University of California at Berkeley.

114 the early 1970s: Samuel Shem, *The House of God* (New York: Dell, 1978), p. 38.

116 care is improved: Timothy B. McCall, "The Impact of Long Working Hours on Resident Physicians," *NEJM*, Vol. 318, No. 12 (March 24, 1988).

116 the hospital money: This study, conducted by Daniel Gottlieb, et. al., appeared in the October 1991 edition of the *Archives of Internal Medicine*; see Lynne Lamberg, "Sleepworking," *American Medical News*, November 6, 1995.

117 getting unduly fatigued: T.F. Deaconson et. al., "Sleep Deprivation and Resident Performance," *JAMA*, Vol. 260 (1988), pp. 1721–1727.

118 a night off: Timothy B. McCall, "Sleep Deprivation and Performance of Residents," letter, *JAMA*, Vol. 261, No. 6 (February 10, 1989).

118 New York State: See Section 405 of the New York State Health Code.

118 114 teaching hospitals: See *The AHA Profile of United States Hospitals,* 1993–4, American Hospital Association, Chicago, 1993, p. 201.

0119 a single shift: See Karen Pallarito, "Experts Still Deliberating Effectiveness of N.Y. Rules Limiting Residents' Hours," *Modern Healthcare,* November 19, 1990.

119 over eighty hours: Information on the process that led to the Bell regulations becoming law was provided by Bertrand Bell, Wayne Osten of the New York State Department of Health, and former New York State Health Commissioner Mark Chassin.

119 million a year: See Kenneth E. Thorpe, "House Staff Supervision and Working Hours: Implications of Regulatory Change in New York State," *JAMA,* Vol. 263, No. 23 (June 20, 1990).

119 million a year: This information was provided by Wayne Osten and Mark Chassin. One reason for the difference between Kenneth Thorpe's $358 million required to implement the Bell regulations, and the reality of $200 million spent is the refusal of the federal government through Medicare and Medicaid to share in the costs of funding the program.

119 most residency programs: Information on the development and passage of the ACGME regulations on hours and supervision was provided by ACGME Executive Director John C. Gienapp. Information on the AMA's development of their rules was provided by Steve Ellwing, staff director of the AMA's resident physician section since 1990. California pediatrician Brian Greenberg also provided information. Currently a member of the board of the California Medical Association, he held several senior positions in the AMA/RPS during the early 1990s. Also see "Memo from the AMA Board of Trustees on Residency/Fellowship Working Conditions and Supervision," *Report KKK,* AMA internal document, June 1991.

120 hours a week: In 1987, the AMA Center for Health Policy Research found that residents were performing resident-related duties for an average of 74.2 hours per week, not counting moonlighting. Interns averaged 85 hours per week for all specialties, and over 100 hours per week for surgical specialties. These hours showed an increase from a previous AMA study done in 1983. See A.B. Silberger et. al., "The Changing Environment of Resident Physicians," *Health Affairs,* Supplement (1988), pp. 121–133. Since 1987, hours have probably decreased slightly as call nights have moved farther apart, but perhaps not as much as many people believe. According to a 1991 survey of resident working conditions sponsored by the AMA, residents spent an average of 57.2 hours per week on call in the hospital—plus the hours they were not on call, though these were not tabulated. (At a very modest eight hours a day working on noncall days, the total weekly hours would easily equal over eighty hours—a figure that is, if true, higher than the average in 1987). In the 1991 survey, surgeons spent an average of 71.4 hours per week on call, easily pushing their total hours over 90 hours. The longest number of hours without sleep in the intern year averaged 38.1 hours for all residents in this study, and 43.5 hours for surgeons. If these survey results are at all accurate, then they contradict the general notion among educators that hours have been going down since the late 1980s. See Steven Daugherty et. al., "Survey of Resident Educational and Working Conditions," *Report to the AMA-ERF* (Chicago: American Medical Association, April, 1991).

122 *uncertain or disagreed:* Joseph Conigliaro, et. al., "Internal Medicine Housestaff and Attending Physician Perceptions of the Impact of the New York State Section 405 Regulations," *Journal of General Internal Medicine,* Volume 8 (September, 1993), p. 502.

123 *a few blatantly:* See Mark Green, *For Whom the "Bell" Tolls: How Hospitals Violate the "Bell" Regulations Governing Resident Working Conditions,* Public Advocate for the City of New York (November 1994).

123 *eighty-hour average:* The handful of residents I interviewed and followed in New York hardly constitute a widespread or scientific sampling, though I was struck by the fact that every resident I spoke with said they have, at times, routinely worked more hours that the regulations stipulate. Many were also only vaguely aware of what, exactly, the maximum hour counts were.

124 *do not, however:* See Green, *For Whom the "Bell" Tolls,* p. 25.

124 *shifts on call:* During this resident's forty-hour stints, there is sometimes little to do if he has no cases, and his patients are being managed by other services.

124 work-week limit: Green, *For Whom the "Bell" Tolls,* p. 7.

124 the state's satisfaction: This is according to New York State investigator Wayne Osten.

124 visited twelve hospitals: See New York State Department of Health, Bureau of Hospital Services, "Resident Regulations Surveillance Status (Surveys of NYC Hospitals with Residency Programs), Calender Year 1993," issued September 30, 1994.

124 least one department: New York State Department of Health, Bureau of Hospital Services, "Resident Regulations Surveillance Status (Surveys of NYC Hospitals with Residency Programs), Calender Year 1992," issued September 30, 1994.

124 twenty-four hospitals: New York State Department of Health, Bureau of Hospital Services, "Resident Regulations Surveillance Status (Surveys of NYC Hospitals with Residency Programs), Calender Year 1991," issued December 30, 1991.

125 twenty-four consecutive hours: New York State Department of Health, Bureau of Hospital Services, "Statement of Deficiencies and Plan of Correction, St. Luke's/Roosevelt Hospital," completed February, 1992, p. 5.

125 $2,000 per violation: This is according to state health department investigator Wayne Osten.

125 of the law: Mark Green, *For Whom the "Bell" Tolls,* p. 25.

126 out of the kitchen: From the film *Bad Medicine?*

126 the old regime: Christine Laine, et. al., "The Impact of a Regulation Restricting Medical House Staff Working Hours on the Quality of Patient Care," *JAMA,* 269:3 (January 20, 1993), pp. 374–378.

126 in patient outcomes: Amalia Kelly, et. al., "The Effect of the New York State Restrictions on Resident Work Hours," *Obstetrics and Gynecology,* 78:3, Part 1 (September, 1991), pp. 468–473.

126 are better rested: See Ibid., and Joseph Conigliaro, et. al., "Internal Medicine House Staff and Attending Physician Perceptions of the Impact of the New York State Section 405 Regulations," *Journal of General Internal Medicine,* Volume 8 (September, 1993).

127 hours a year: See Juliet Schor, "Americans Work Too Hard," Op-Ed, *New York Times,* July 12, 1991.

128 put to rest?: R. Carlson, "Residency Work Hours: Will the Controversy Be Put to Rest?," *Texas Medicine*, 87(3) (March, 1991), pp. 38–50.

CHAPTER 6: SCUT AND THE 20% SOLUTION

129 X ray quest: Cindy Williams and Mrs. Morro are pseudonyms.

132 understaffed ancillary services: According to ACGME officials, overusing residents for noneducational service work is one of the most prevalent violations of their code. Further proof comes from New York, where hospitals are paid a total of $200 million a year, in part to pay for ancillary personnel hired to take on non-physician duties performed by residents before the Bell Regulations limited their hours.

132 felt excited, proud: Shem, *The House of God,* pp. 53–54.

132 of a rabbit: The Oxford Dictionary of English Etymology, ed. C.T. Onions (Oxford: Oxford University Press, 1983 edition), p. 803.

133 and patient transport: Robert J. Schwarta, et. al., "Guidelines for Surgical Residents' Working Hours: Intent vs. Reality," *Archives of Surgery,* Volume 127 (July, 1992), pp. 778–779.

133 time to scut: Ibid. Other studies have rated "scut" at anywhere from 17% to 62%. For example, see Robert S.A. Haywood, et. al., "A Phenomenology of Scut," *Annals of Internal Medicine,* 115:5 (September 1, 1991), pp. 372–376; N. Lurie, et al., "How Do House Officers Spend Their Nights? A Time Study of Internal Medicine House Staff on Call," *NEJM,* 320 (1989), pp. 1673–1677.

134 them by residents: Letter from Catherine A. Horan, ACGME Administrator to Edward A. Iannuccilli, Director of Medical Education, Rhode Island Hospital, June 29, 1994. This letter announced the ACGME's decision to give Rhode Island Hospital a "favorable" rating for continued accreditation as a teaching hospital. This rating was issued with three "comments," including the following: "It is unclear whether blood drawing services are adequately provided in a manner appropriate for and consistent with educational objectives, patient care and cost-effectiveness. Residents reported that these services were cut back in the evening and late-night hours in response to budgetary limitations experienced by the institution's pathology department." CFO John Schibler said he would investigate the blood drawing situation to determine if there was a problem.

136 *to organize orders:* See Testimony of Luise Weinstein, *Zion v. New York Hospital,* New York State Supreme Court, Manhattan, 1994. Peter Crean, one of Weinstein's lawyers during the Zion case, verified that Weinstein was tending to patients' routine needs, and writing notes during this period. Many of these patients were very ill, said Crean, but none were in acute distress.

136 *last several hundred:* Numerous time studies of how residents spend their days have found that they spend long hours writing notes. Most suggest a range of time from about a quarter to a third of a resident's call day spent on this activity. For instance, see N. Lurie, et. al., "How Do House Officers Spend Their Nights?" Also see F.J. Kroboth, et. al., "Amount and Distribution of Residents Working Hours," *Academic Medicine,* 65:542 (1990). These numbers correlate with what several educators told me.

136 *of the night:* Spending hour after hour writing notes and performing scut also reduces the time residents spend with patients. Kroboth and his colleagues report that only 12% of daytime activity and 37% of nighttime activity for interns was spent directly with patients. See Kroboth, "Amount and Distribution of Residents Working Hours."

137 *the bottom line:* In 1989, when New York enacted the Bell Regulations, the State Department of Health agreed to help compensate for fewer resident hours by providing money to hire more ancillary care—and more residents. Since then, the state and private insurers have spent about $200 million a year to implement the regulations. However, according to a 1994 study released by the New York City Public Advocate's Office, at least part of this money has gone into the general budgets of hospitals, and has not always gone to hire more ancillary personnel. Likewise, not all the state money allocated to pay attendings to comply with the Bell Regulations' provision to increase supervision has been directly linked to attendings actually working more hours as supervisors. See Mark Green, *For Whom the "Bell" Tolls: How Hospitals Violate the "Bell" Regulations Governing Resident Working Conditions,* Office of the Public Advocate for the City of New York (November, 1994).

137 *his surgical residents:* This is Dr. Frank Spencer of New York University, who told his audience at an AMA seminar in 1991 that to fund backup personnel for ten residents working reduced hours, it would cost $200,000. The few published studies attempting to analyze the relationship between reducing resident hours and the need to increase ancillary services suggest that Spencer is right—costs will increase. "The number of full-time equivalent physician's assistants or nurse practitioners needed to replace one resident would have increased costs by more than 300%," writes Jonathon Klein in one study. Klein, "Resident Education, Work Hours, and Supervision: Time for Change," *Journal of Pediatrics,* 116:3 (March, 1990), pp. 484–486.

137 *hospital a dime:* Actually, residents do produce substantial income for hospitals, performing services and attracting funding from the government through Medicare.

138 *him Mr. Jacobs:* Mr. Jacobs is a pseudonym.

138 *for their hospital:* See David Ewing Duncan, "Anatomy of a Medical Bill," *Life,* December, 1993, pp. 15–18; and "Anatomy of a Hospital Bill," *ABC Nightline,* November 16, 1993. These numbers are based on actual bills the author reviewed from several hospitals, interviews with hospital financial officers, and various studies.

139 *$5,000 to $12,000:* See Duncan, "Anatomy of a Medical Bill," for salary figures.

139 *taxes—plus benefits:* This is based on a PGY5 getting a $32,500 annual salary, and working an average of 98 hours per week—the national average for a surgical resident—with three weeks vacation. A PGY1 in this hospital earns about $30,000 a year.

139 *$148,000 a year:* See *American Medical News,* January 10, 1994, p. 1.

140 *in most programs:* See *AAMC Data Book,* January, 1994, table G1.

140 *some 30 percent:* Ibid., Table E1.

140 *a decade earlier:* Ibid., Table E4.

141 *to nine years:* Congress now defers student loans for graduate students for only two years. In cases of extreme hardship, loan payments are deferred for three years. Currently, those residents who began their training on or before July, 1993 are allowed to

defer during their entire training period; residents beginning after this date are subject to the new rules. Source: Steve Ellwing, staff director of the AMA's resident physician section.

141 *constant, 1970 dollars:* These figures were presented in a speech by James Stockman, Chairman, Department of Pediatrics, Northwestern University Medical School. See Stockman, notes, pg. 5. According to AAMC data, PGYIs in 1971 were paid an average of $26,522 in 1992 dollars, adjusted for inflation. In 1992, PGYIs were actually paid $28,618. See *AAMC Data Book,* January, 1994, Tables G1 and L1.

141 *as a PGY5:* The median income for surgeons in 1992 was $206,000. See *American Medical News,* January 10, 1994, p. 1. Numerous physicians were also polled by the author to determine how much a starting surgeon might expect to be paid. Salaries differ considerably according to location and employer.

141 *is over $550,000.* Source: Medical Group Management Association, as reported in the *New York Times,* November, 1993.

141 *her current income:* the median income for a family practitioner in 1992 was $100,000. See *American Medical News,* January 10, 1994, p. 1. Numerous physicians were also polled by the author to determine how much a starting family practitioner might expect to be paid. Salaries differ considerably according to location and employer.

143 *legitimate hospital expense:* See John E. Wennberg, et. al., "Finding Equilibrium in U.S. Physician Supply," *Health Affairs* (summer, 1993), pp. 89–103; also see Meaghan Jared Partners, Inc. and Arthur Anderson & Co., *Analysis of Medical Education Costs: Volume 1: Final Report,* January 10, 1991; and Jeffrey J. Stoddard, et. al., "Graduate Medical Education Reform: Service Transition Costs." *JAMA,* 272:1 (July 6, 1994), pp. 53–58. In 1993, researchers writing in *The Journal of Medicine* estimated that the annual house staff substitution costs amounted to between $58,000 and $77,000 per resident. This means that if teaching hospitals in the United States reduced residency slots by 25 percent, or roughly 23,200, it would cost them $1.4 billion to $1.8 billion to replace residents with ancillary personnel. See C. Parenti and N. Lurie, "Are things different in the light of day? A time study of internal medicine house staff days," *American Journal of Medicine,* 94 (6) (June, 1993), pp. 654-58.

143 *for by attendings:* See Thomas L. Simmer, et. al., "A Random-
ized, Controlled Trial of an Attending Staff Service in General
Internal Medicine," *Medical Care,* Volume 29, Number 7 (Supplement) (July, 1991).

143 *cost of care:* Robert M. McNamara, et. al., "Cost of Care in the
Emergency Department: Impact of an Emergency Medicine Residency Program," *Annals of Emergency Medicine,* 21:8 (August,
1992), pp. 957–959.

143 *in total revenues:* See "Analysis of Medical Education Costs,"
Rhode Island Hospital, December 17, 1993, p. 2–2.

143 *similar-sized hospitals:* Ibid. Rhode Island used data similar to
its own collected at several other academic medical centers.

144 *amounts, exist elsewhere:* Ibid. The hospitals used in Rhode
Island's analysis were redacted in the study before being provided
to the author.

144 *year of 1984:* Information about HCFA funding of graduate medical education was provided to the author in a series of phone
interviews with Tzvi Hefter, director of HCFA's Division of Hospital Services, which administers Medicare's program on funding
graduate medical education.

144 *$90,000 per resident:* See "Analysis of Medical Education
Costs," Rhode Island Hospital, p. 2–2. These amounts are combined direct and indirect Medicare payments. Medicare makes
payments to teaching hospitals under these two categories: 1)
direct payments, which support direct costs such as resident
salaries, benefits, faculty salaries, the building and maintenance
of on-call rooms, and so forth; and 2) indirect payments, which
are designed to compensate hospitals for what they claim are
additional costs accrued by having trainees in house—costs in
additional tests, longer lengths of stay for patients, and the fact
that most teaching hospitals support sizable populations of uninsured and indigent patients.

145 *$45,000 per resident:* This number was provided by the office of
Nelson Ford, Chief Financial Officer for Georgetown University
Hospital in Washington, D.C.

145 *for residency programs:* Source: Tzvi Hefter, director of Division
of Hospital Services, Medicare, HCFA. In 1995, direct Medicare
payments for graduate medical education was projected to be
$1.49 billion—an amount determined by a hospital's purported

"direct" costs as determined in 1984, plus an annual increase based on the Consumer Price Index. Indirect payments are expected to total $4.58 billion, and are based on a formula that takes into account a complicated statistical analysis of factors contributing to higher costs in teaching hospitals and the ratio of residents to beds. [Sources: Tzvi Hefter of HCFA; also C. Anthony Ross, "Medicare Support of Medical Education," *Health Affairs*, 7:2, Supplement, (1988), pp. 158–159]. Medicare payments represented about 35% of the total revenues to support residencies in America. The remainder came mostly from patient billing. [Source: *American Medical News*, August 7, 1995].

145 *residents as possible:* James M. Carl and Ronald J. Knaus, "A Primer on Graduate Medical Education Financing," *JAOA*, Volume 93, Number 10 (October, 1993), p. 1058.

145 *in measured costs:* Herbert S. Diamond, et. al., "An Analysis of the Cost and Revenue of an Expanded Medical Residency," *Journal of General Internal Medicine*, Volume 8 (November, 1993), pp. 614-618. The authors of this study make the point that profits from reimbursement was not a motivation for expanding their residency.

146 *of American Medicine:* Starr, *The Social Transformation of American Medicine*, pp. 359–360.

146 *their residency slots:* See "Results of the National Resident Matching Program for 1995," *Academic Medicine*, Volume 69, Number 6 (June, 1995), pp. 508–509.

146 *3,000 from abroad:* Ibid. For the number of teaching hospitals, see *Hospital Statistics*, American Hospital Association, 1993–4, p. 200.

147 *power is moonlighting:* In 1987, the AMA reported that more than one in three residents said they regularly moonlighted. See A.B. Silberger et. al., "The Changing Environment of Resident Physicians," *Health Affairs*, Supplement (1988), p. 128.

147 *or withheld accreditation:* See "Accreditor Proposes Tighter Rein on Residency Programs," *American Medical News*, March 27, 1995.

147 *inner-city facilities:* "Hospitals Stripped of Credentials: Training Program Axed," *Newsday*, August 12, 1994, p. A12. According to Dr. Stephen Weseley, Associate Dean for Graduate Medical Education at New York Medical College, which administered the

orthopedic programs at Lincoln and Metropolitan, the college has applied to the ACGME to start a new orthopedic residency based at two other hospitals in their system—St. Vincent's Hospital in New York and Westchester County Medical Center in Valhalla, New York. The college has no plans to start new programs in Lincoln or Metropolitan.

147 *precedence over service:* See "Accreditor Proposes Tighter Rein on Residency Programs," *American Medical News,* March 27, 1995.

CHAPTER 7: FOR THE LOVE OF MEDICINE

149 *her medical degree:* Carol Tisch is a pseudonym.

157 *to medical school?:* Alan B. Cohen, et. al., "Young Physicians and the Future of the Medical Profession," *Health Affairs,* Winter, 1990, pp. 142–143.

157 *their own children:* "A Measure of Satisfaction," *Hippocrates* questionnaire, February, 1994. See "Anatomy of a Burnout," *Hippocrates,* April, 1994, p. 40.

157 *of their jobs:* "Can You Care Too Much?" *Hippocrates* survey, April, 1994.

157 *roles as physicians:* "A Measure of Satisfaction," *Hippocrates* questionnaire, February, 1994. See "Anatomy of a Burnout," *Hippocrates,* April, 1994, p. 40.

158 *in Dothan, Alabama:* The story of Mark Stafford originally appeared in *Hippocrates* in a slightly different form. See David Ewing Duncan, "Compassion Fatigue: Can You Care Too Much?" *Hippocrates,* February, 1994, pp. 34–41.

159 *ill cancer patients:* The story of William Porter originally appeared in *Hippocrates,* February, 1994.

161 *of their situation:* See Thomas Delbanco, et. al., "Clinical Crossroads: An Invitation," *JAMA,* Volume 274, Number 1 (July 5, 1995), pp. 76–77.

162 *42,000 in 1974:* See *AAMC Data Book,* January, 1994, Table B1.

162 *to come by:* David A. Shaywitz, "The Bedside Profession," *The New York Times,* editorial, July 10, 1995.

163 *the East Coast:* Randy Gaines is a pseudonym. Other names and places associated with his story have been changed or altered slightly.

166 *a fair characterization:* Bill Moyers, *Healing and the Mind,* (New York: Doubleday, 1993), p. 7.

166 *being a healer:* Ibid., pp. 22–23.

CHAPTER 8: DO THE KIND THING FIRST

168 Epigram: *suffer with me:* Anatole Broyard, "The Patient Examines the Doctor," *Intoxicated by My Illness And Other Writings on Life and Death* (New York: Fawcett Columbine, 1992), p. 44.

168 *Mr. Ivan Maximov:* This is a pseudonym.

169 *When Pete Nichols:* Pete Nichols is a pseudonym.

170 *calmly taking notes: The Gross Clinic,* painting by Thomas Eakins, 1875.

171 *asking anyone's permission:* See Gina Kolata, "Hospitals Use Bodies of Dead for Practice," *New York Times,* December 15, 1995. The study was conducted by Dr. Jeffrey P. Burns of the New England Medical Center in Boston; Dr. Robert D. Truog of Children's Hospital in Boston; and Frank Reardon, a lawyer. The study was published in *The New England Journal of Medicine.*

175 *be too great:* Broyard, "The Patient Examines the Doctor," p. 49.

176 *arrogance and unkindness:* From the "Physician" section of the *Hippocratic Corpus,* c. fourth and fifth centuries, B.C.; quoted from *Ethics in Medicine: Historic Perspectives and Contemporary Concerns,* ed. Stanley Joel Riser et. al. (Cambridge, MA: MIT Press, 1977), p. 7.

176 *do it first:* William Osler, quoted in Paul B. Beeson, "On Becoming a Clinician," *On Doctoring,* ed. Richard Reynolds and John Stone (New York: Simon & Schuster, 1991), p. 178.

176 *least two years:* See Daniel Goleman, "Doctors Find Comfort Is a Potent Medicine," *New York Times,* November 26, 1991.

176 *for their fractures:* See James J. Strain, et. al., "Cost offset from a psychiatric consultation with elderly hip fracture patients," *The American Journal of Psychiatry,* 148 (August, 1991), pp. 1044–9.

176 *a heart attack:* See Goleman, "Doctors Find Comfort Is a Potent Medicine," *New York Times,* November 26, 1991.

176 *for medical problems:* Ibid.

177 *of the physician:* From the "Precepts" section of the *Hippocratic Corpus,* c. fourth and fifth centuries, BC.; quoted from *Ethics in Medicine,* p. 5.

177 *such ideas folklore:* Marcia Angell, "Disease as a reflection of the psyche," editorial, *NEJM,* 312:24 (June 13, 1985), pp. 1570–2.

177 *describing their illnesses:* See Stanley Joel Reiser, *Medicine and the Reign of Technology* (New York: Cambridge University Press, 1978), p. 196. Also see Reiser for general information about the rise of the scientific method in clinical medicine.

178 *those still open:* See Abraham Flexner, *Medical Education in the U.S. and Canada: A Report to the Carnegie Foundation for the Advancement of Teaching* (Carnegie Foundation for the Advancement of Teaching: New York, 1910).

178 *peculiarly its own:* Abraham Flexner, *Universities: American, English, German* (New York: Oxford University Press, 1930), p. 21.

178 *to human suffering:* Abraham Flexner, *Medical Education: A Comparative Study,* (New York: MacMillan, 1925), pp. 11–12.

179 *and their griefs:* William Osler, "The Leaven of Science," [1894], from *Counsels and Ideals from the Writings of William Osler* (New York: Houghton, Mifflin & Co., 1905), p. 128.

179 *it is funny:* Broyard, "The Patient Examines His Doctor," 46.

179 *than the doctor:* Osler, "The Student Life," [1905], from *Counsels and Ideals from the Writings of William Osler,* pp. 111–112.

179 *rules of evidence:* Edmund Pellegrino, "The Reconciliation of Technology and Humanism: A Flexnerian Task 75 Years Later," *Flexner: 75 Years Later, A Current Comment on Medical Education,* ed. Charles Vevier (New York: University Press of America, 1987), p. 103.

179 *fondly, as poets:* See Lawrence K. Altman, "Physicians Endorse More Humanities For Premed Students," *New York Times,* November 14, 1989. Altman, a physician, cites a 1986 study by Drs. David Fraser and Leah Smith of Swarthmore College that showed only 14% of physicians they surveyed, whose undergraduate experiences spanned the years 1955 to 1982, had majored in the humanities.

179 *enroll more poets:* Comments from Edmund Pellegrino and Tom Delbanco.

182 *My Own Medicine:* Quoted from *The Doctor,* Touchstone Pictures, 1992; a film based on Edward Rosenbaum's *A Taste of My Own Medicine: When the Doctor Is the Patient* (New York: Random House, 1988).

183 *to congenital defects:* William Osler, *Aequanimitas* (New York: McGraw-Hill, 1932).

184 *says Tom Delbanco:* Delbanco and his colleagues have studied
doctor-patient interactions by polling both on their attitudes
toward the other. "One of our unpleasant findings is," he says,
"that patients with chronic illnesses encounter far more problems in communicating with doctors than do patients who are
not so sick." See Paul D. Cleary, et. al., "Patients Evaluate Their
Hospital Care: A National Survey," *Health Affairs* (winter, 1991),
pp. 254–67; and Thomas L. Delbanco, "Enriching the Doctor-
Patient Relationship by Inviting the Patient's Perspective,"
Annals of Internal Medicine, 116:5, pp. 414–8.

184 *of all four: Curriculum Directory,* 1994–95, Association of
American Medical Colleges, Washington, D.C.

184 *science and physiology:* In a poll *Hippocrates* conducted as
recently as the summer of 1995, 68 percent of young doctors said
they agreed strongly or somewhat with the statement: "Medical
school does not train doctors to deal with the emotional needs of
patients. How strongly do you agree?" *Hippocrates,* Novem-
ber/December, 1995, p. 41.

185 *a respectful attitude:* Tom L. Beauchamp and James F. Childress,
Principles of Biomedical Ethics, Fourth Edition, (New York:
Oxford University Press, 1994), p. 125.

186 *a Vandyke beard:* Bob Zapita is a pseudonym.

CHAPTER 9: AN INTERN FOREVER

188 Epigram. *their long existence: Program and Policies: The Interne
Council of America.* (New York: The Interne Council of America, 1940), p. 1.

189 *pick her up:* Testimony of Sidney Zion, from *Zion vs. New York
Hospital, Raymond Sherman, Luise Weinstein, Gregory Stone,
and Maurice Leonard,* New York Supreme Court, New York
City. The trial ran from November 10, 1995 to February 6, 1996.
Quotes and descriptions from the *Zion vs. New York Hospital*
trial come from the author's notes while attending the trial,
Court TV broadcasts, and trial transcripts. Unless otherwise
indicated, facts related to the Zion case and trial come from *Zion
vs. New York Hospital* testimony and court documents. The latter include such items as Libby Zion's medical chart and autopsy

report. The author has also reviewed other key documents in a case that spans over a decade, and has generated thousands of pages of material. These include testimonies and opinions gathered during investigations of the Zion case conducted or initiated by the grand jury convened in Manhattan in 1985, the State Board for Professional Medical Conduct, the Regents Review Committee of The University of the State of New York, and the New York State Commissioner of Health. Other sources include legal documents prepared by lawyers in the civil case; M.A. Farber, "Who Killed Libby Zion?" *Vanity Fair*, December, 1988, pp. 190–195, 214–228; and Natalie Robins, *Every Patient's Nightmare: The Girl Who Died Twice: The Libby Zion Case and the Hidden Hazards of Hospitals* (New York: Delacorte, 1995). The author also interviewed lawyers representing the two sides in the Zion civil trial.

189 *daughter is dead?:* Robins, *Every Patient's Nightmare*, 28–29. This dialogue was verified by Sidney Zion.

189 *was Shloft gezunt:* Testimony of Sidney Zion, *Zion vs. New York Hospital.*

189 *Ray, what happened:* Ibid.

189 *could have done:* To my knowledge, Ray Sherman has not disputed the basic content of these two calls on March 5, 1984.

189 *was a fluke:* Testimony of Sidney Zion, *Zion vs. New York Hospital.*

190 *during this call:* See Robins, 138–139.

190 *talking about this:* Testimony of Sidney Zion, *Zion vs. New York Hospital.*

190 *negative in another:* See autopsy record of Libby Zion, Office of Chief Medical Examiner, City of New York, signed by Jon S. Pearl, M.D., 5/18/84. The autopsy was performed on March 6, 1984.

190 *blood collected:* See ibid. and Robins, 121–122 for details about Zion's blood tests.

190 *swab material:* See autopsy record of Libby Zion, Office of Chief Medical Examiner, City of New York, Report from the toxicology laboratory, statement signed by Milton L. Bastos, Director of Laboratory, 5/8/84. The record states: "SWABS: Trace of cocaine detected by (RI)—not enough material for confirmation by (TLC)." RI and TLC are tests used to identify cocaine.

190 *negative for cocaine:* Autopsy record of Libby Zion, Office of Chief Medical Examiner, City of New York. Tests conducted on Libby's postmortem liver and bile also came out negative. Cocaine metabolizes quickly once consumed, though trace elements remain for up to 48 hours. Libby Zion's postmortem blood, which came out negative for cocaine, was drawn about 27 hours after her death. To confuse matters further was a subsequent blood test run by the chief examiner's office in August, 1984 on Libby's antemortem blood, which had tested positive in one test for cocaine shortly after Libby's death. In August, five months later, this same blood tested negative for cocaine using the same test. See Report from the Office of the Chief Medical Examiner, City of New York, Supplementary Report, 8/27/84. During the trial, Zion's expert witnesses argued that the evidence for cocaine was at best inconclusive, and that other plausible theories existed to explain her death. They also questioned the timing of Libby's condition, which remained essentially unchanged during her first four hours in the hospital, but apparently changed dramatically sometime during the three hours leading up to her code at 6:40 a.m. on March 5, some seven hours after her admission. Could cocaine consumed at 8 or 9 p.m. the evening before have caused such a sudden worsening many hours later? Not surprisingly, the experts were divided on this and virtually every other question regarding cocaine, with the hospital and its lawyers and experts contending that the autopsy records suggest the possibility of cocaine, and that Libby's symptoms were consistent with a bad cocaine reaction. Yet no one has offered indisputable evidence that cocaine is what killed Libby Zion.

190 *acute pneumonitis:* Autopsy record of Libby Zion, signed by Jon S. Pearl, M.D., 5/18/84. Dr. Pearl also mentions that Libby Zion was taking Nardil. He does not explain what is meant by "toxic agitation," or what the source of the toxicity might be. Later, Dr. Elliot Gross, the chief medical examiner, speculated that Libby died of "hemorrhagic pneumonia," which usually occurs as a result of bacterial infection. Later still, other experts suggested that the hemorrhaging may have been caused by trauma inflicted during the attempt to resuscitate Libby. See Robins, p. 61.

191 *New York Hospital:* See Robins, *The Girl Who Died Twice,* p.

152. Numerous experts have testified and analyzed Libby Zion's condition the night she died, with some concluding that the thrashing, high temperature, high white blood cell count, and other indicators are consistent with a serious bacterial infection. Others testified that even small amounts of cocaine can cause thrashing, and in very rare cases, lead to death. While a patient at New York Hospital, Libby was not screened for cocaine or other illicit drugs that might have settled the question of drug use while Zion was still alive. One tentative diagnosis, according to charts written by the R2, Greg Stone, was a possible viral infection and what he described as "hysterical symptoms." Stone and others have also said that Libby's agitation that night was at least in part voluntary, since she would stop for a time when asked to. Stone and Weinstein both considered a bacterial infection, but apparently ruled it out, since she was never administered intravenous antibiotics. State Medical Examiner Dr. Jon S. Pearl notes that "the patient had signs and symptoms of sepsis." See Autopsy record of Libby Zion, signed by Jon S. Pearl, M.D., 5/18/84.

191 *as a teenager:* See Robins, *The Girl Who Died Twice*, pp. 79-88.

191 *night in 1984:* Even one of New York Hospital's attorneys, Peter Crean, called the evidence that Libby Zion ingested cocaine on March 4, 1984, "circumstantial," though he still believes "the evidence presents a very strong case," even if no one actually saw Libby take cocaine that night.

191 *also a consideration:* Admission note of Dr. Luise Weinstein, March 5, 1984, from the medical chart of Libby Zion.

191 *in the trial:* Sidney Zion might have added the issue of the doctor's handling of Libby's suspected drug use to his list of negligence counts, but opted not to, saying it was not necessary given his insistence that she did not take drugs that night.

191 *of her treatment:* Hospital attorney Peter Crean said that a toxicological blood test had been ordered for Libby, to be done later on the morning of March 5.

192 *count of 18,200:* Admission note, March 4, 1984, from medical chart of Libby Zion.

192 *for Libby Zion:* Dr. Sherman insists that Greg Stone did not mention Demerol during his phone conversations with Stone on the night of March 4-5, 1984.

192 *for criminal indictment:* "Report of the Fourth Grand Jury for the April/May Term of 1986 Concerning the Care and Treatment of a Patient and the Supervision of Interns and Junior Residents at a Hospital in New York County," The New York Supreme Court, December 31, 1986.

193 *danger to patients:* "Report of the Fourth Grand Jury," Preface, p. 2–3. New York Hospital and others have criticized the grand jury report as basing its findings on faulty information.

193 *graduate medical education:* Jonathan Klein, "Resident Education, Work Hours, and Supervision: Time for Change," *Journal of Pediatrics* (March, 1990), p. 484.

195 *treat Libby Zion:* Verdict Sheet, *Zion vs. New York Hospital,* delivered on February 6, 1995.

195 *allowed to consider:* The civil suit jury could only judge the specifics of this case, based on what the judge allowed, what was specifically germane, and what the lawyers from both sides were able and willing to produce. A grand jury can look at any and all evidence it pleases, issuing judgments and statements on virtually anything it deems worthy.

196 *a physician's approval:* See "Stipulation and Order OC-87-17" (with respect to New York Hospital), taken by the New York State Department of Health with respect to alleged violations of state public health laws, codes, and regulations, signed by David Axelrod, State Commissioner of Health, and Raymond Sweeney, Director of the Office of Health Systems Management, March 12, 17, 18, 1987.

196 *not admit guilt:* Ibid., p. 3. According to medical reporter M.A. Farber, New York Hospital claimed that it admitted to these procedural lapses to avoid a long case that might hold up approval from the state for new construction at the hospital. See M.A. Farber, "Who Killed Libby Zion?" *Vanity Fair,* December, 1988, p. 194.

196 *revisit this issue:* Decision of Judge Elliott Wilkes regarding motions in *Zion vs. New York Hospital,* New York Supreme Court, City of New York, May 1, 1996.

198 *on the wards:* Information on Luise Weinstein comes from her testimony at various hearings and at *Zion vs. New York Hospital;* additional information comes from interviews with people who know her. The author requested an interview with Dr.

Weinstein through New York Hospital, but was told she does not wish to discuss the Zion case or talk to the media. "Luise is a private person," commented Weinstein's lawyer, Peter Crean, when author Natalie Robins approached him about speaking with Dr. Weinstein.

199 *conduct in 1989:* See "Statement of Charges in the Matters of Gregg W. Stone, M.D. and Luise L. Weinstein, M.D.," State of New York, Department of Health, State Board for Professional Medical Conduct, August 31, 1989.

199 *staff and others:* David Axelrod, "Commissioner's Recommendation to the New York Board of Regents, In the Matters of Gregg W. Stone, M.D. and Luise L. Weinstein, M.D.," State of New York, Department of Health, State Board for Professional Medical Conduct, November 14, 1989, p. 2.

200 *L. Weinstein:* Quoted from Libby Zion's medical chart, New York Hospital. "Death note" entered by Luise Weinstein on March 5, 1984.

202 *evaluate the patient:* Testimony of Luise Weinstein, *Zion vs. New York Hospital.*

203 *at all times:* Joseph Hayes says that every night an attending, or an R6 or R7, rounds to check on every patient on his service.

204 *from their effort:* "The Public Gains From the Zion Case," *New York Times,* editorial, February 8, 1995.

205 *and the plaintiff:* Lelia B. Helms and Charles M. Helms, "Forty Years of Litigation Involving Residents and Their Training: II. Malpractice Issues," *Academic Medicine,* Vol. 66, No. 12 (December, 1991).

205 *the United States:* This number is speculative. It comes from David U. Himmelstein and Steffie Woolhandler, *The National Health Program Book,* (Monroe, ME: Common Courage Press 1994), p. 139. Himmelstein and Woolhandler are respected physicians and researchers at Cambridge Hospital in Massachusetts. Their number of lawsuits comes from extrapolating the data from T.A. Brennan et. al., "Incidence of adverse events and negligence in hospitalized patients: results of the Harvard Medical Practice Study I," *NEJM,* 324 (1991), 370–376.

205 *Dr. Connie Guion:* See Carol Lopate, *Women in Medicine* (Baltimore: The Johns Hopkins Press, 1968), pp. 105–106.

206 *since Guion's day:* For information and sources on the history of

residency reform in America, see Robert G. Harmon, "Intern and Resident Organizations in the United States: 1934–1977," *Milbank Memorial Fund Quarterly/Health and Society*, 56:4 (1978), pp. 500–530. Also see Lily M. Hoffman, "House Staff Activism: The Emergence of Patient-Care Demands," *Journal of Health Politics, Policy and Law* 7:2 (Summer, 1982), pp. 421–439.

206 *Greater New York:* Harmon, "Intern and Resident Organizations," p. 501.

206 *compensation for interns:* Ibid., pp. 501, 504.

207 *and Communist affiliations:* Ibid., p. 504.

207 *up to 100 percent:* Ibid., pp. 506–507.

208 *the job action:* "3,000 Doctors Strike at 23 Hospitals," *New York Post*, March 17, 1975.

208 *to newspaper accounts:* A special bulletin published in 1975 by the Committee of Interns and Residents (CIR) in New York City reprinted virtually every article written on the New York strike. Copy provided by CIR.

208 *the picket lines:* Quoted in Lucinda Franks, "NYU Hospital Interns Bar Strike, Saying They Won't 'Forsake' Patients," *New York Times*, March 19, 1975.

209 *for 17,108 positions:* Paul Jolly, "Medical Education in the United States," *Health Affairs*, 7:2, Supplement (1988), p. 152.

209 *medicine went unfilled:* Between 1985 and 1990, the number of medical school graduates entering internal medicine dropped 27%, from 3884 students to 2829 students. In 1990, 58% of categorical (traditional) medicine positions and 44% of primary care positions went unfilled. P.R. Kletke et. al., "Changes in the Supply of Internists: The Internal Medicine Population from 1978 to 1998," *Annals of Internal Medicine*, 107 (1987), pp. 93–100.

210 *Medicine in 1991:* Bruce C. Vladeck, "Where Do We Go from Here?" *Bulletin of the New York Academy of Medicine*, 67:4 (July-August), 1991.

210 *of Internal Medicine:* James P. Nolan and Thomas S. Inui, "Tinkering or Real Reform? The Choice Is Ours," *Annals of Internal Medicine*, 116:12 (Part 2) (June 15, 1992), pp. 1042–1045.

210 *drugs and alcohol:* See Mark D. Schwartz et. al., "Medical Student Interest in Internal Medicine: Initial Report of the Society of General Internal Medicine Interest Group Survey on Factors Influencing Career Choice in Internal Medicine," *Annals of*

Internal Medicine, 114:1 (January 1, 1991), pp. 6–11. Also see Julia E. MacMurray, et. al., "The Attractiveness of Internal Medicine: A Qualitative Analysis of the Experiences of Female and Male Medical Students," *Annals of Internal Medicine,* (October 15, 1993), pp. 812–818.

210 *the spring match:* This was confirmed by John Stobo, then Chief of Medicine at Johns Hopkins. The match is the system by which resident candidates are offered positions with residency programs. It works by having programs and candidates list their top choices, which are then matched by a computer.

210 *with the match:* John Stobo says that one reason Hopkins did not match in 1991 was because they listed fewer than usual applicants. Stobo explained that to fill their 30 or so positions, they usually list 120 names. In 1991, he said, they listed fewer, thinking they would get more of their top choices to match with them.

212 *codes and regulations:* "Memo from the AMA Board of Trustees on Residency/Fellowship Working Conditions and Supervision," *Report KKK,* AMA internal document, June, 1991.

212 *four-week period:* Ibid., p. 1

212 *and other issues:* Ibid., pp. 1–2.

213 *pursuing government intervention:* Other sources put the number of states as high as sixteen.

213 *mandatory accreditation requirements:* See "Essentials of Accredited Residencies in Graduate Medical Education," Section II of *Essentials and Information 1995–1996,* Accreditation Council for Graduate Medical Education, (Chicago: American Medical Association, 1995), pp. 11–278. Historic information was provided by John Gienapp, executive director of the ACGME, and Steve Ellwing, staff director for the AMA's resident physician section, during phone interviews.

214 *California and Massachusetts:* For California, personal communication and documents provided by Brian Greenberg, member of the board of the California Medical Association; for Massachusetts, see "Massachusetts: Union Contracts Best Bet for Hours Reform?" Article draft prepared by the CIR, Boston chapter.

214 *for some time:* Personal communication with Laura Morelock, a lead researcher at Johns Hopkins for the New York study investigating the outcome of the Bell Regulations.

214 *supervision and hours:* For instance, see the New York state Department of Health Incident Reports; also see Mark Green, *For Whom the "Bell" Tolls: How Hospitals Violate the "Bell" Regulations Governing Resident Working Conditions,* Public Advocate for the City of New York, November 1994.

216 *unwanted sexual advances.* "Disputes Between Medical Supervisors and Trainees," Council Report by the Council on Ethical and Judicial Affairs, AMA, *JAMA,* Vol. 227, No. 23, December 21, 1994, pp. 1861–1865. This report reviews several surveys of residents on the subject of abuse. Also see excerpts from the "Resident Forum" in *JAMA,* including: Kirsti Dyer, "Grievance Issues and Resident Abuse: Resources Available," *JAMA,* Vol. 274, No. 1, July 5, 1995, p. 4; and "Filing Complaints Against Residency Programs, Parts I and II," *JAMA,* Vol. 273, No. 21, June 7, 1995, and Vol. 273, No. 22, June 14, 1995.

217 *call James Dooley:* James Dooley is a pseudonym.

CHAPTER 10: COMMON SENSE: A BLUEPRINT FOR CHANGE

222 Epigram. *secret of revolutions:* Antoine Saint-Just, *Speech to French National Convention, 1793.* Found in *A New Dictionary of Quotations on Historical Principles from Ancient and Modern Sources,* ed. H.L. Mencken (New York, Alfred A. Knopf, 1987), p. 1033.

223 *would be home:* The no-call system, says Most and others, needs to be refined in terms of when shifts begin and end, what happens when there are too few or too many patients, and so forth. For instance, Most says patient admissions are heaviest in late afternoon and early evening, which suggests that a resident's "day" may need to start and end later than it does now.

224 *his work well:* Aristotle, *Nicomachean Ethics,* tr. Martin Ostwald (Indianapolis, IN: Bobbs-Merrill 1962), p. 43.

227 *night float system:* Henry W. Foster Jr., and Vicki L. Seltzer, "Accommodating to Restrictions on Resident's Working Hours," *Academic Medicine,* 66:2 (February, 1991), pp. 94–97.

227 *care or education:* Other changes include dual residencies, where two residents take one slot, with one working, say, one month, and the other the next month. Some programs and hospi-

tals also make an effort to hire husbands and wives together, if possible.

228 *physicians and surgeons:* Bertrand M. Bell, "Greenhorns in White," editorial, *New York Times*, February 9, 1995.

228 *classroom and lab:* For instance, see Eugene A. Foster, "Long Term Follow-Up of an Alternative Medical Curriculum," *Academic Medicine*, 69:6 (June, 1994), pp. 501–506; John Thompson et. al., "The Accelerated Internal Medicine Program at the University of Kentucky," *Annals of Internal Medicine*, 116:12 (Part 2) (June 15, 1992), pp. 1084–1087; C. Briggs-Style, et. al., "The Effects of Early Patient Contact: The Student's Perspective," Proceedings of the Twenty-Ninth Annual Conference on Research in Medical Education, *Academic Medicine*, 65:Supplement (September, 1990), pp. S33–S34.

228 *other outpatient settings: 1994 Directory of Family Practice Programs*, American Academy of Family Physicians (Kansas City, MO).

228 *care resident's year:* In 1992, during a retreat of the Association of Professors of Medicine sponsored by the Robert Wood Johnson Foundation, participants called for "Changes in the current three-year residency that would result in 50% of educational time being spent in ambulatory care locations." Harold J. Fallon, "Residency Reform: A Perspective from the Association of Professors of Medicine," *Annals of Internal Medicine*, 116:12 (Part 2) (June 15, 1992).

229 *into primary care:* Esther B. Fein, "More Young Doctors Forsake Specialty for General Practice," *New York Times*, Monday, October 16, 1995, p. 1.

229 *did not decline:* See *American Medical News*, January 22/29, 1996, p.1.

229 *clinics, or CCs:* See Marilyn C. Dumont-Driscoll, "Pediatric Resident's Continuity Clinics: How Are We Really Doing?" *Pediatrics*, Vol. 96, No. 4 (October, 1995), p. 616.

230 *to fifty-six hours:* See "Doctors' Hours Cut—Hip, Hip," *The Lancet*, Volume 336 (December 22/29, 1990), pp. 1543–1545.

230 *to seventy-two hours:* See "England Imposes 72-Hour Limit on Residents," *JAMA*, Vol. 265 (May 22, 1991 and May 29, 1991).

230 *of sixty hours:* See Canadian Association of Internes and Residents, Ontario Province Rules and Regulations, p. 18.

230 *hours a week:* See "Doctors' Hours Cut—Hip, Hip," *The Lancet,* p. 1543

230 *on the wards:* See John Corboy and Peter Herbison, "Trainee interns: education and service roles," *New Zealand Medical Journal,* 106 (965) (October 13, 1993), pp. 431–2. In 1985, after voluntary controls failed to reduce hours in New Zealand, government-imposed financial penalties worked—by requiring that programs pay steep overtime wages to residents.

230 *resident workweek:* Ibid.

232 *redress, if indicated:* Strengthening the ACGME's investigative methods would also help; currently, a staff of seventeen full- and part-time evaluators visit an average of three institutions a week, always with ample warning. Typically, they meet with residency program directors, selected faculty, and as many residents as possible in a battery of one- or two-day meetings. They do not routinely take tours of facilities or investigate specific programs unless they have received a legitimate complaint from a resident or faculty member. Otherwise, the accreditation process—which is underwritten by the AMA, the American Hospital Association, and other medical organizations—depends on volumes of forms asking questions about everything from numbers of patients treated by pediatric residents to how many overnight beds are available for trainees. One wonders what the investigators would see if they appeared unannounced and followed residents as I have through overnight calls—a process that is currently beyond the mission and budget of the ACGME. Sources: *Assuring the Quality of Medical Care,* ACGME brochure, and a phone interview with Steven Nestler, an ACGME official based in Chicago.

232 *not be painless:* Timothy McCall, "No Turning Back: A Blueprint for Residency Reform," editorial, *JAMA,* 261:6 (February 10, 1989), pp. 909–10.

237 *health care policy:* See Eggert R.W., Parkinson, "Preventive medicine and health system reform: improving physician education, training, and practice," *JAMA,* Vol. 272, 1994, pp. 688–693. Also see Thomas Clancy, et al., "A Call for Health Policy Education in the Medical School Curriculum," *JAMA,* Vol. 274, No. 13 (October 4, 1995), pp. 1084–1085.

237 *well as healers:* J.C. Cantor, et. al., "Preparedness for practice:

young physicians' views of their professional education," *JAMA*, Vol. 270, 1993, pp. 1035–1040.

238 *at teaching hospitals: The New York Times*, editorial, May 15, 1995.

238 *close it down:* AMA/RPS Report: "Residents Working With Managed Care Problems," Introduced by Dexanne B. Clohan, *Report C*, 1994 AMA Interim Meeting.

238 *to do so:* This information was provided by Marty Heath, a spokesperson for Timberlawn hospital.

239 *less experienced—doctors:* See Elisabeth Rosenthal "Deaths After Surgery Prompt an Inquiry at L.I. Hospital," *The New York Times*, August 1, 1995, p. A1.

239 *next few years: American Medical News*, August 7, 1995. In the fall of 1995, a national panal of health care experts, the Pew Health Professions Commission, sponsored by the Pew Charitable Trusts, released recommendations to scale back the number of medical school slots by 20 to 25 percent over the next ten years. They also recommended sharply reducing the number of foreign medical graduates allowed to train in United States residency programs. The commission noted that many experts believe an optimal number of physicians is about 150 per 100,000 population, far below the current 240 per 100,000. See Esther B. Fein, "Medical Schools are Urged to Cut Admissions by 20%," *The New York Times*, November 17, 1995.

0239 *health care budget:* Deborah Shelton, "Los Angeles County Faces Massive Public Health Cuts," *American Medical News*, August 7, 1995. Steve Ellwing of the AMA, and John Gienapp of the ACGME cited managed care's reduced cash flow to hospitals as a major factor in the county health care system's financial woes.

240 *realities of medicine:* See Richard Saltus, "Beth Israel, Harvard join to train MDs in home, clinic," *The Boston Globe*, January 3, 1996.

For descriptions of residency rankings, see "Ranks, Titles, and Terms" at the beginning of the book.

AAMC: Association of Academic Medical Centers.

Academic Medical Center: A complex that includes one or more hospitals affiliated with a medical school, with a full complement of residency programs.

ACGME: Accreditation Council of Graduate Medical Education, the body that officially accredits residency programs.

Admission: a patient entering the hospital, whether through the emergency room, or at the request of a personal physician.

AMA: American Medical Association.

Aneurysm: a ballooning out of a vessel, especially an artery, before it bursts.

Angioplasty: Inserting a tiny balloon into the heart to force open a stuck valve.

Attendings: physicians finished with their training who either are on the staff of a teaching hospital, or have a private practice and admitting privileges.

Attending Rounds: Each month on the wards and in the O.R.'s, an attending from the teaching faculty is assigned to oversee teams of residents. Legally responsible for the patients on their team, these ward attendings spend an hour or two each day, usually late in the morning, hearing reports and plans from team members on patients. Usually, rounds include a session in a conference room and at the bedside of patients being cared for by the team.

Black Cloud: A resident having bad luck.

Boxoid A patient likely to die, i.e., likely to be boxed.

BUN: Blood Urea Nitrogen; an indirect measure of heart failure.

CAT-scan: Also called a CT-scan, for computed tomography devices that use computers and low-radiation X rays to take images of a patient's internal anatomy.

Call (Also "on call" and "call night"): A period of time, usually a day and an overnight when a resident stays in the hospital to admit new patients, take care of patients already admitted, and supervise more junior trainees. A traditional call lasts 36 hours.

Cap: A limit placed on the number of patients a resident can admit during a single call night.

Chem 7: A battery of standard blood chemistry tests.

Citizen: A patient considered normal, who talks, is educated, and insured; as opposed to a "noncitizen," who is a drug addict, a homeless drunk, etc.

Code (also "code blue" or "code red"): the term used on a hospital overhead speaker to summon emergency teams to resuscitate a patient in cardiac arrest.

Cross-cover: When a resident on call covers patients belonging to residents on his or her team who are not on call.

CVP: Central Venous Pressure, the pressure in the vein feeding directly into the heart.

Defibrillator: A machine used to attempt to shock a heart back into normal rhythm or to start it again when it has stopped.

DNR: Do Not Resuscitate. A legal order signed by a patient or close relation ordering that heroic measures such as codes or intubation not be attempted due to the terminal nature of the illness.

EKG: A readout of a patient's heartbeat as measured by an EKG monitor.

Epinephrine: A drug that stimulates the autonomic nervous system, it is used to assist in resuscitating a victim of cardiac arrest.

Fellow: A physician in training who has completed a basic residency, and is now training as a specialist.

Foley Catheter: A tube put into the bladder through the urethra to assure flow of urine.

GI: Gastro-Intestinal, pertaining to organs located in the abdomen.

HCFA: Health Care Finance Administration, an entity in the U.S. Department of Health and Human Services that oversees Medicare.

House Staff: Interns and residents in a particular hospital.

HMO: Health Maintenance Organization. An entity that manages health care payments for large pools of people, often by contract with an employer, and often at a discount compared to traditional insurance plans.

Iatrogenic: Injuries caused by the actions or attitude of physicians or from treatment received as a patient in a hospital.

I.C.U.: Intensive Care Unit. Variations include S.I.C.U. (Surgical Intensive Care Unit), M.I.C.U. (Medical Intensive Care Unit), C.C.U. (Cardiac Care Unit), etc.

Intubated: Inserting a rubber tube through the mouth and down into the trachea, which is used to artificially respirate a patient. Patients can also be intubated by placing a plastic tube directly in the trachea, which is attached to a breathing machine called a ventilator.

I.V.: Intravenous, inside a vein, an I.V. line is a tube inserted into a vein via a needle to inject fluids and drugs directly into a patient's blood system.

Managed Care: A nonspecific term that describes a recent movement in health care delivery toward reducing costs by restricting procedures and access to specialists.

M & M: Morbidity and Mortality; a regularly scheduled conference attended by most house staff and faculty in which mistakes and unexpected outcomes are aired.

MI (also a "farc"): Myocardial infarction, a heart attack.

MICU: Medical Intensive Care Unit.

Nasogastric Tube (NG Tube): A narrow plastic tube inserted through the nose and down the esophagus to the stomach, used to suction out fluid to check for internal bleeding.

Neuro: Neurology. The medical specialty dealing with the brain and nervous system.

Night Float: A resident assigned to cover the wards at night, and/or to take admissions overnight, so that on call residents can get caught up on their work, or sleep.

Note: Entries made by a physician or nurse into a patient's medical chart.

Orders: Requests made by physicians and nurses for tests and services to be performed on patients, for example, an X Ray or a drug to be administered.

Ortho: Orthopedics, the surgical specialty dealing with bones and joints.

PGY 1, PGY 2, etc.: Post Graduate Year 1, Post Graduate Year 2, etc. One's standing in terms of years in their residency program.

Ray Rounds: Checking X rays with a radiologist.

Rounds: Meetings convened by residents and/or attendings to discuss patients. Can also refer to an individual physician checking up on patients as in "personal rounds."

RPS: Resident Physicians Section, an AMA organization with elected delegates and officers established to provide a voice for residents within the AMA.

Scut: Any onerous or repetitive task; particularly those menial tasks performed by residents that do not require an M.D. and don't contribute to education, such as drawing blood and chasing down X rays.

Septic: An infection of the blood, leading to infection of a major organ, and to septic shock, in which the blood pressure falls.

SICU: Surgical Intensive Care Unit.

STAT: At once, immediately.

Step-Down Unit: A step down from intensive care, where patients are monitored, but are not as critical as those in the ICU. Also called a *pasture*, where patients are weaned from a respirator.

Teaching Hospital: 1,223 hospitals in the United States that have at least one residency program.

Toxic: Refers to the introduction of drugs or bacteria that act like poison to damage major organs. Also refers to a physician who is very stressed.

Triage: Sorting out patients according to severity of injury or disease, so that the most severe are attended to first.

Triple Threat: The traditional imperative among medical educators to excel at being clinicians, researchers, and teachers.

Unit (The Unit): any intensive care unit.

Ventilator: A machine that breaths for a patient unable to breath on their own.

ACKNOWLEDGMENTS

Hundreds of people have contributed to this book, and to my experience of living among and studying not only residents but the art and science of medicine. No one deserves more thanks than my wife, who has tolerated and supported what amounts to my "residency" researching, reporting, and writing this book. My children, Sander, Danielle, and Alexander, also were unusually tolerant while their dad was away in the field, or holed up writing on weekends and evenings.

Also a warm thanks to my friends and advisors—Steve Vicchio, for his constant and unflagging support and encouragement, and his insistence on my keeping true to my intentions; Lonny Hecker, who read the manuscript and wrote a touching and highly useful appraisal; and TK, who all but ordered me to complete this project.

I could never have written this book without the urging and affection of Charles Scribner, III, his cohort in editing and congeniality, Hamilton Cain; and Jennifer Chen. Also, thanks to Mel Berger, agent extraordinaire, and his assistant, Claudia Cross; to Steve Petranek, who has always believed in me; and Gerry Marzorati and Colin Harrison, who got the ball rolling.

I am not able to list all the residents who helped me by name, but they know who they are. I admire their courage and wish to change things for the better. Thanks to Jim Stern, Frank Luccia, Gregory Kuhn, Janice Walker, Randolph Martin, Benjamin Frain, Bill Kidd, Claude Kelly, Greg Maines, Rebecca Patchin, Fiona Bayne, Rich Ferrara, Steve Jones, Geena Carlson, Ben Rollins, James Dooley, Cindy Williams, Peg Miller, Myriam Jones, Carol Tisch, Judy Linger, Laurie McKeown, Steve Thornquist, Randy Gaines, Jim Hargrove, Pete Nichols, and dozens of others who allowed me to speak to them and live among them. (Note: some of these names are pseudonyms, as identified in the reference notes.)

I am not entirely sure how educators and physicians I worked with will receive this book. I'm hoping they will understand that I tried my best to stay true to the facts, and to fairly present all sides. Special thanks to Dominique Tamaro, Al Most, Bertrand Bell, Tom

Delbanco, John Stobo, John Potts, Dan Brock, Steve Bergman, Edmund Pellegrino, Bill Frishman, Robert Meyer, Lucian Leape, Brian Greenberg, Jennifer Jeremiah, William Hazel, Edward Iannuccilli, Robert Nye, Joseph Hayes, John-Henry Pfifferling, Nassir Ghaemi, and Colin Stern. A few educators are not listed, but they perhaps know who they are—to them, I hope they understand a husband's anguish, and will read this book with a fresh eye.

Thanks also to Steve Ellwing, John Gienapp, Tzvi Hefter, Wayne Osten, Mark Levy, Merrill Mitler, Sidney Zion, Thomas Moore, Judy Livingstone, Frank Bensel, Peter Crean, and Beth Karas.

I also thank my two assistants, Denise Hawkins and Amy Dean—you are the best.

Of course, any errors or wrong-headed thinking is entirely my own fault.